Holographic Reprocessing for Healing Trauma, Abuse, and Maltreatment

T0372877

Holographic Reprocessing for Healing Trauma, Abuse, and Maltreatment addresses root causes of symptoms that develop as a result of traumatic experience including repetitive cycling of trauma called experiential holograms. Holographic reprocessing offers strategies to sharpen conceptualization and to effect change. Using the observer vantage point, people can consider context and contributing factors to holistically reappraise their perceptions and meaning of the past. Holographic reprocessing also engages experiential learning and corrective emotional experiences for deep transformation. This book outlines a step-by-step process to 1) identify experiential holograms, 2) consider reappraisals, and 3) reprocess using an imagery-based procedure of visiting one's younger self. This novel approach is integrative, easily tailored to individual needs, and well-grounded in theory. It can be applied to a variety of traumatic experiences including interpersonal abuse, moral injury, medical, and military trauma. Numerous outcome studies support a growing evidence-base for the efficacy of this treatment. This book is an indispensable guide for trauma clinicians.

Lori S. Katz, Ph.D., is a clinical psychologist specializing in the treatment of trauma. She received the Sarah Haley Memorial Award for Clinical Excellence from the International Society of Traumatic Stress Studies. She is the author of *Holographic Reprocessing: A Cognitive-Experiential Psychotherapy for the Treatment of Trauma* (2005), *Warrior Renew: Healing from Military Sexual Trauma* (2014), and *Treating Military Sexual Trauma* (2015).

Holographic Reprocessing for Healing Trauma, Abuse, and Maltreatment

Lori S. Katz

Foreword by Andrei Novac, M.D.

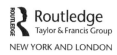
Routledge
Taylor & Francis Group

NEW YORK AND LONDON

Cover image © Getty Images

First published 2024
by Routledge
605 Third Avenue, New York, NY 10158

and by Routledge
4 Park Square, Milton Park, Abingdon, Oxon OX14 4RN

Routledge is an imprint of the Taylor & Francis Group, an informa business

© 2024 Lori S. Katz

Access the Support Material: resourcecentre.routledge.com/books/
9781032121727

Library of Congress Cataloging-in-Publication Data
Names: Katz, Lori S., 1963- author.
Title: Holographic reprocessing for healing trauma, abuse, and maltreatment
/ Lori S. Katz, Ph.D.
Description: New York, NY : Routledge, 2024. | Includes bibliographical
references and index. |
Identifiers: LCCN 2023018425 (print) | LCCN 2023018426 (ebook) |
Subjects: LCSH: Psychic trauma--Treatment. | Cognitive-experiential
psychotherapy.
Classification: LCC RC552.P67 K383 2024 (print) |
LCC RC552.P67 (ebook) | DDC 616.85/21--dc23/eng/20230724
LC record available at https://lccn.loc.gov/2023018425
LC ebook record available at https://lccn.loc.gov/2023018426

ISBN: 978-1-032-12173-4 (hbk)
ISBN: 978-1-032-12172-7 (pbk)
ISBN: 978-1-003-22342-9 (ebk)

DOI: 10.4324/9781003223429

Typeset in Sabon
by Taylor & Francis Books

Contents

Illustrations

Figures

Tables

Disclaimer

This book is intended for gender-neutral audiences. As such, the words "they" and "them" have been substituted for singular pronouns, unless addressing a specific gender-identified person. Although case examples are included, specific details and identifying information have been significantly altered to protect client privacy. Some cases are a compilation of more than one client, again to protect people's privacy.

This book is intended as a guide for professionals. As with any treatment manual, clinical judgment supersedes protocol. The author and publisher assume no responsibility for how this information is used. This book is not a substitute for professional mental health services.

About the author

Lori S. Katz, Ph.D. is a clinical psychologist specializing in the treatment of trauma during her career working for the Department of Veterans Affairs. She was the recipient of the International Society of Traumatic Stress Studies (ISTSS), Sarah Haley award for clinical excellence. She has published several books: *Holographic Reprocessing: A Cognitive-Experiential Psychotherapy for the Treatment of Trauma* (2005), *Warrior Renew: Healing from Military Sexual Trauma* (2014), and *Treating Military Sexual Trauma* (2015).

Foreword

Andrei Novac, M.D., DFAPA

It is with great honor that I have undertaken the task of preparing this foreword for what I consider a major leap forward in providing a healing context for human trauma. Dr. Lori Katz has dedicated her talent, her vast clinical and research skills, and her personal life experience in creating a healing space that has improved the lives of many patients.

It is then inspiring to be part of the publication of *Holographic Reprocessing for Healing Trauma, Abuse, and Maltreatment*. The release of this book is meaningful in the context of recent progress in our understanding of traumatic stress. Noteworthy, since the 1970s, following the early contributions in psychoanalysis to treatment of trauma, new therapies have emerged with the purpose of producing better results in less time and at a lesser cost. However, in time, past therapeutic approaches have faced the reality of dropout rates, adverse effects, and need for modification.

Holographic reprocessing is a technique that deeply assesses the entire individual in the context of trauma. Such treatment results not only in reduction of symptoms and processing of traumatic intrusions, but also in significant personal and psychosocial growth.

In order to delve into the ramifications of the workings of holographic reprocessing, I would like to recapitulate the basics of how trauma changes memory, the body, and our stories. Previously, I have referred to trauma as a virtual impact between a human being and an event (Novac, 2003). Both humans and life events are equal players in the equation of the trauma impact, contributing with their own specifics: the individual's past experiences, personal predispositions, family history; the specifics of the event, e.g., proximity, timing, intensity, social context. For this reason, the outcome is highly unpredictable. Then, one of the main difficulties in addressing trauma lies in its myriad variable outcomes.

A large body of research has been validated regarding the neuroscience of trauma. When in the 1970s James McGaugh discovered that catecholamines (adrenaline/noradrenaline) have a direct memory consolidation effect, he opened the door to further understand the impact of human trauma

(McGaugh, 1983). With its excessive release of catecholamines at the time of the *traumatic impact or repeated impacts,* trauma will lead to a rapid consolidation of raw, unprocessed memories of a traumatic experience: events, perceptions, fears.

We have since learned that unlike routine everyday experiences that are processed through the dominant left hemisphere of the brain, and in particular the speech areas, traumatic memories of adverse experiences are stored predominantly in the right hemisphere of the brain. These are very complex and painful and become rapidly consolidated as unprocessed raw material, similar to loud static (Rauch et al., 1996). Unprocessed consolidated memories tend to be spontaneously reactivated, by subliminal reminders in the environment. Such reactivations are highly distressing and further reactivate the entire catecholamine system. This, in turn, tends to further re-consolidate and amplify the original trauma. A viciously repeated perfect storm is created, and with each repetition of the cycle, the distress and horror of the trauma is duly re-experienced and re-imprinted. That re-imprinting reaches the deep levels of implicit scaffolding of our autobiographical memory.

For humans, stories about themselves and others are quintessential. Self-narratives, the stories that we tell about ourselves, are based on the subtype of episodic memory, the autobiographical memory. Under normal circumstances, many memories are retold, some in semi-chronological order. Out of myriad life events, only certain memories remain in place, deeply imprinted, to become a cast in a person's autobiography. This is due to an implicit memory scaffolding initiated early in life. Previously, I have referred to this part of implicit memory as Identity Narrative (IdN) (Novac et al., 2017a., 2017b, 2019a, 2019b, 2021). In this context, traumatic stress is now understood as a deeply carved-in process that becomes part of who we are. This is a self-maintained process that includes high experiences of body sensations and mental torment. This is often followed by traumatic enactment in relationships, which constitutes behaviors for survival of future encounters with trauma. Such enactment also becomes part of a new trauma-specific implicit self-narrative.

Viewed from inside, for a victim of trauma, the world is never the same again. Research has also revealed that such fundamental changes are accompanied by a resetting of the hypothalamic pituitary axis, with changes in the corticosteroid response, which gravely limits a person's future neurophysiological coping with adversities (Yehuda, 1993). These are not known to be self-maintained mechanisms, but instead, these actions spread over years and decades from the original trauma(s). As has been documented by van der Kolk (2015), the body keeps score of the trauma, and I would submit that the body and the mind change their personal story or personal narrative.

Beginning with her first book in 2005, *Holographic Reprocessing: A Cognitive-Experiential Psychotherapy for the Treatment of Trauma,* Dr.

Katz has embarked on a continuous journey of developing a new evidence-based treatment for trauma. This latest endeavor, *Holographic Reprocessing for Healing Trauma, Abuse, and Maltreatment* adds the experience of almost two decades of work with holographic reprocessing. Placed within a spectrum that ranges from dynamic therapies to cognitive techniques of healing, holographic reprocessing is meant to transform the entire person, irrespective of the individual manifestation of a particular trauma.

Holographic reprocessing is effective in reducing suffering, preventing comorbidity of PTSD, and alleviating the horror of living with constant intrusions from the trauma. This is accomplished through several stages in the treatment process, which include strategies in attaining emotional regulation; self-soothing; and awareness and contemplation. Change is further facilitated by two main factors: discovering a context as a new way to perceive the past; imagery reprocessing, a way to revisit a younger self and rewrite a traumatic script. The benefits of treatment remain active long-term and continue to provide an implicit memory repair mechanism to work towards a post-traumatic renewal of one's self, what has been referred to as posttraumatic growth.

Holographic reprocessing has a unique place in trauma treatment. By using specific techniques that emphasize a reprocessing of multilevel memories from unprocessed intrusions to self-perception and body memory, holographic reprocessing further aims to rework implicit narratives. By acknowledging that imagery, affect and sensation are the "royal roads" to an individual's self and autobiography. Holographic reprocessing modifies the traumatized self in a holistic manner. Holographic reprocessing helps us rewrite a life story. Those new life scripts reopen doors to allow life to continue and unfold in a context of personal, social, and spiritual freedom. Such freedom and liberty to choose constitutes the moral and holistic legacy of holographic reprocessing.

Andrei Novac, M.D., DFAPA
Diplomate, American Board of Psychiatry and Neurology
Clinical Professor of Psychiatry
University of California at Irvine

References

Katz, L. S. (2005). *Holographic reprocessing: A cognitive-experiential psychotherapy for the treatment of trauma.* New York: Brunner-Routledge.

McGaugh, J. L. (1983). Preserving the presence of the past. Hormonal influence on memory storage. *American Psychologist, 39,* 161–173. doi:10.1037/0003-066X.38.2.161.

Novac, A. (2003). Global and social considerations, Special report (guest editor) *Psychiatric Times,* 20(4):33.

Novac, A, Bota, R. G., & Blinder, B. J. (2017a). Identity narrative density: Preliminary findings from scoring emotional valence of autobiographical events. *Bulletin of the Menninger Clinic,* 81(4), 299–313.

Novac, A., Tuttle, M. C., Bota R, Yau J. B., & Blinder B.J. (2017b) Identity and autobiographical narratives: Towards an integrated concept of personal history in psychiatry. *Mental Health and Family Medicine*, 13, 625–636.

Novac, A., Tuttle, M. C., & Blinder, B. J. (2019a). Identity Narrative and its role in bio-logical survival: Implications for child and adolescent psychotherapy. *Journal of Infant, Child, and Adolescent Psychotherapy*, 18(2), 155–184.

Novac, A., Tuttle, M. C., Bota, R. G., & Blinder, B. J. (2019b). Identity narrative as an unconscious scaffold for human autobiography. In: *New studies and research in multidisciplinary fields*, pp. 106–112. Rome: European Centre for Science Education and Research (EUSER) and Mediterranean Centre for Science Education and Research (MCSER).

Novac, A., Zahn, C., & Blinder, B. J. (2021). Identity narrative, group and individual narratives and their role in social stability: A multidisciplinary approach. *Group Analysis*.

Rauch, S. L., van der Kolk, B., Fisler, R, Alpert, M., Orr, S. P., Savage, C.R., Fischman, A. J., Jenike, M. A., & Pitman, R. K. (1996). A Symptom provocation study of posttraumatic stress disorder using positron emission tomography and script-driven imagery. *Archives of General Psychiatry*, 53(5), 380–387. doi:10.1001/archpsyc.1996.01830050014003.

van der Kolk, B. (2015). *The body keeps the score: Brain, mind, and body in the health of trauma*. Penguin publishing group.

Yehuda, R. (1993). Stress and glucocorticoid. *Science*, 275, 1662–1663.

Preface

I have a distinct memory of waiting in line to enter my third-grade class-room. I was eight years old amongst a group of about 20 other eight-year-old girls, all wearing green plaid uniforms and white knee-high socks. We looked similar, yet there were clear social distinctions of who was most popular and who was not. Those who were popular claimed it as so—self-declared, and asserted their rank, were territorial, and some were a bit mean. Maybe they felt entitled, or maybe they just wanted to protect their status. Others who appeared uneasy and insecure thought they were less than the popular ones. They believed the falsehood. I was in a unique status of neutrality—not in either group, yet able to interact with both. What I realized that day, was that objectively those deemed popular were really no different than anyone else. It was artificial, a construction, something cre-ated, and everyone acted as if it was the truth. My distinct memory was sharing my epiphany out loud. I basically said that friendships were choices and it (their coalitions) didn't have to be that way. Then we filed into the classroom as if nothing happened. It was a non-event. Even writing this now, the words don't convey my thought process, but for me it was a grand epiphany, and quite memorable.

I was intrigued by what was objective truth, and what was a constructed truth. People perceive things about themselves and other people, and these stories or narratives are encoded in one's implicit system, outside of their conscious awareness. For efficiency, the belief, like a snapshot, becomes the default setting: "I'm like this; they are like that." They react to their own and other people's constructions as if they were truth, and because they believe them, it *is* their truth. People live in their own perceived realities. Their perceptions are based on what they have experienced. It is what they know; and therefore, their reality, even if not objectively true. In most cases, these perceptions are based on limited information, and are only part of the picture, but not the whole picture.

Perhaps there are some along a narcissistic or sociopathic continuum that claim and believe perceptions of reality to fuel their desired inflated sense of self-importance. They may or may not have the capacity to imagine how others feel. Regardless, they don't seem to care. They may perceive others as insignificant or objects to be used for self-gain. Furthermore, they may be motivated to shape or control other's perceptions to match their own. There are others, without the capacity to imagine an objective reality such as those with psychosis or those in severe mental states. People in the aforementioned categories may be so engrossed in their own subjective reality that they lack motivation, desire, and possibly capacity to consider an objective reality or anything outside of their self-perceptions.

But the majority of humanity actively perceives their experiences and weaves together a coherent narrative of their lives. Most are motivated by basic needs of self-esteem, autonomy, and a desire to emotionally connect with others. They have the ability to imagine how others might feel and have the capacity for empathy. However, due to emotional distress or dysregulation secondary from traumatic experiences, their perceptions have been altered and their processing has been halted. Ensuing trauma-based beliefs become encoded in the implicit system. This is the basis for developing experiential holograms which influence thoughts, feelings, and behaviors. Experiential holograms filter perceptions, like wearing virtual reality goggles, where life is viewed through a trauma-lens. This becomes the default setting for anticipating, interpreting, and responding to life experiences as if they could be potential replications of past trauma. Relevant to this book, people who may be struggling with life lived through a trauma-lens, may benefit from this treatment. By considering context from an objective vantage point, they may gain insight. Ultimately, they may release negative affect, and expand, rewrite, and shift their trauma-based perceptions to increased self-compassion, and empathy.

Back in third grade, I could see two realities. Like seeing a magic trick as magic, and seeing the technique of what's behind the magic, simultaneously. Ever since, I have been driven by the simple question, "Why is it so?" Not surprisingly, I pursued academic studies seeking to understand our psycho-social functioning. At the University of Massachusetts, I worked under Dr. Seymour Epstein, who mentored and taught me cognitive-experiential theory (CET). But once again I found myself in a liminal space. I opted for a double major completing a research and clinical degree. I was not in one major, but both. I did not belong to either camp, theoretical orientation, or social clique. There is a gift of not belonging. It affords the benefit of critical evaluation from the observer vantage point. With knowledge of CET as a global theory of personality, I was intrigued to explore the essence of healing across various therapies.

It wasn't until the early 1990s when I was immersed in clinical work, that holographic reprocessing was conceived. I came across the book *The Holographic Universe* (Talbot, 1991) which gave me the language to describe the cognitive-emotional-social patterns that I had been observing in my clients. They were like holograms, living in repetitive patterns that were very real to the client, but objectively not real at all. I first introduced my ideas to the scientific community in a poster session for the 1999 American Psychological Association (APA) annual conference. The first article was published in 2001 in the APA journal, *Psychotherapy* and in 2005, the first book on holographic reprocessing was published by Brunner-Routledge (Katz, 2005). About 18 years later, it seems worthy to reflect on how knowledge about this treatment has evolved. What changes have been made, and what areas need further inquiry?

Holographic reprocessing is currently an emerging evidence-based clinical practice. I've been contacted by clinicians (from various countries) who have been successfully using this approach. This supports positive practical application—with real-world anecdotal accounts. However, it is difficult to track how many people are actually using holographic reprocessing, and with unknown fidelity to the model.

Thus, systematic evaluation is necessary to closely monitor and test the efficacy of the treatment. It requires years of concerted effort to objectively evaluate treatment outcomes. With much gratitude, several researchers have chosen to put forth this effort to evaluate holographic reprocessing and have done so independent of influence from me. While I have conducted a few studies with a team of providers, a true test of a treatment is the research conducted by those with no invested interest in the outcomes.

An evolution of the treatment, based on holographic reprocessing, is the development of a specialized treatment for military sexual trauma and interpersonal trauma across the lifespan, called *Warrior Renew: Healing from military sexual trauma* (Katz, 2014). It is delivered as a group treatment targeting salient topics related to sexual trauma such as self-blame and resentment due to lack of closure. Eight pragmatic trials have demonstrated significant reduction in symptoms. Two more studies are in progress including a randomized clinical trial funded by the United States Department of Defense.

At this time, a total of 17 outcome studies have been conducted on holographic reprocessing including 14 based on randomized clinical trials demonstrating effective outcomes, and 8 published studies on warrior renew. The aggregate of these studies supports a growing evidence base, demonstrating significant reduction of symptoms (e.g., depression, anxiety, negative thinking), improvement of positive factors (e.g., self-esteem, quality of life, cognitive flexibility, traumatic growth), and with low dropout rates. As Najavits (2015) noted, evaluating a treatment should include not only measuring the reduction of symptoms but also examining attrition to determine if the treatment is acceptable and feasible. Thus far, these treatments are associated with remarkably low dropout and with positive feedback from participants.

Also, when evaluating the efficacy of a treatment, it is prudent to test it with different treatment populations with diverse human factors, delivered by a variety of therapists, and offered in a variety of formats. Holographic reprocessing has been utilized with survivors of military and non-military sexual trauma; those with combat related moral injury, depression, and posttraumatic stress disorder (PTSD: APA 2013), those in recovery from substance abuse, and with diverse and gender inclusive samples in the United States. It has also been studied with people with cancer; women with depression from recent divorce with and without infidelity; women with a recent suicide attempt, and adolescent males with mixed traumas in Iran. The warrior renew program has been delivered as part of a 12-week intensive outpatient program, as an outpatient group, as a brief 8-session treatment delivered in primary care both in-person and over video in a telehealth format, and was used as the curriculum in a five-day retreat. Evidence collected from diverse studies continues to accumulate supporting the efficacy, feasibility, and practical application of holographic reprocessing treatment to diverse populations delivered in flexible formats.

With continued practice and teaching of the model, developments have emerged since 2005. Several new metaphors and clinical strategies are used to help efficiently explain concepts by appealing to the experiential system of the mind. Examples are using *virtual reality goggles*, and addressing *blueprints* to explain the influence of experiential holograms. Another example is the concept of a *meta-reframe* to shift perceptions and consider context. These new advancements will be discussed in this book.

One of the basic components of holographic reprocessing is to find out why a person is having symptoms and behaving in their particular way. It seeks to help make sense of people's experience. As stated, the experiential hologram resides outside conscious awareness, although it automatically influences people's thoughts, feelings, and behaviors. They may struggle with repetitive consequences. Their effort to climb out of the hole only digs it deeper. It is a unique and bold task of this treatment to inquire *why*. It challenges therapists to enter the client's experiential reality, work to make connections, and find explanations even when one does not seem apparent. This is in essence what holographic reprocessing is about—identifying, reappraising, and releasing limited perceptions to allow natural healing to occur. It utilizes toggling between being in the experience, to observing oneself in the experience. As an observer, people can see context, release pain, gain insight, and imagine completing communications. By targeting root causes, it expedites healing, resulting in permanent, lasting change.

Continued research is needed to further our understanding of experiential holograms and how to best implement this model of care. One area for continued growth is to delve deeper into typologies of experiential holograms, as there may be as many as there are emotional patterns. Another growth point is to expand offerings for training and supervision/consultation for those interested in implementing holographic reprocessing. This is a goal for the next ten years with the mission to empower clinicians with tools so they can give their clients a way to free themselves from painful experiential holograms. I believe I share a vision, with other clinicians and healers, to help as many people as possible release their pain and embrace their optimal functioning. The hope is to help people reconnect to their hearts with compassion, forgiveness, and joy.

Lori S. Katz, Ph.D.

Acknowledgements

This book comes to fruition with the influence and support of many. It begins with a thank you to Seymour Epstein, Ph.D. for his mentorship and cognitive-experiential theory, which has been a guiding foundation for my work. I have much gratitude to Geta Cojucar, M.S., for her determination, optimism, and unwavering support. Sincere thanks to Wayne Thomas, Sr. for his continued support and encouragement, and to my dear friend Gina Jensen, L.C.S.W. who urged me to write this book. Thank you to my esteemed colleague Andrei Novac, M.D., for writing an impactful foreword. I am tremendously grateful for Amanda Wood, Ph.D. for spear-heading an enormous task of conducting a randomized clinical trial. Thanks to Nicole Myers, M.D., for her strong desire to make a difference. Many thanks to the researchers who studied holographic reprocessing and whose work is referenced in this book. And thank you to the many others who have shaped my thinking along the way. Finally, it is with great respect that I acknowledge my patients. I marvel at their courage and resilience. I thank them all.

Foundation for holographic reprocessing

Part I

Foundation for holographic
reprocessing

Chapter 1

Introduction to holographic reprocessing

This chapter begins with a case example illustrating how experiential holograms, based on past experiences, filter how people respond to life circumstances. It is an example of people engaging in everyday life, showing the subtle yet pervasive nature of experiential holograms. This chapter provides a brief overview of the book content. It also introduces cognitive-experiential theory and compares it to the major theories of psychotherapy namely, psychodynamic and cognitive-behavioral theories.

Case example: Abby and Trina

Abby and Trina worked together as waitresses at a busy restaurant. Abby was relatively new to this restaurant, but was a seasoned waitress and had a long history of working at different locations. Over the course of a couple of months, Abby noticed Trina was a bit aloof and irritable towards her. Finally, Abby asked Trina if she was ok. Trina shrugged. With prodding, she agreed to talk.

She told Abby that she dreaded taking shifts with her for concerns that Abby would leave early and she would have to pick up the last tables. She felt that Abby was unreliable. Abby was shocked and asked what she was referring to. Trina told her that on the day before Thanksgiving, Abby left early and Trina was swamped. Abby was apologetic and quickly offered to take an extra shift for Trina. Trina appreciated talking about it and her efforts to make things right.

However, Abby was bothered by the interaction. First of all, she never leaves early, and secondly, why would Trina hold on to that incident for over two months? Furthermore, Abby is on late shift four days a week and frequently gets swamped with the last table. Abby looked at her calendar and saw that she was on scheduled sick leave the day before Thanksgiving and had put it on the shared work calendar in two places. She felt vindicated and told Trina about it the next day. Trina was grateful that Abby didn't actually leave, but still blamed Abby because she didn't put it in the right spot on the calendar.

DOI: 10.4324/9781003223429-2

Now Abby was upset. She felt falsely accused and was annoyed that Trina assumed the worst about her. Trina said she was ok with Abby, but inside still dreaded working with her. Abby and Trina are both reasonable rational people. Both believed their reactions were justified. But even after discussing this relatively minor misunderstanding, why are they both still upset? Why are they both cautious about having to work together? Likely they are responding to experiential holograms, or emotional patterns based on their past experiences with others:

Trina holds deep resentments about taking care of her younger siblings and household chores while her mother was preoccupied with men and alcohol. She is particularly sensitive to feeling that she has to be responsible for others who did not/or do not do their jobs. Abby has a history of being criticized, falsely accused, and punished for things that she did not do. She is quick to reject those who reject her. To Abby an accusation of not "being good enough" shakes her to her core.

Experiential holograms are learned from past experiences and become the filter through which people anticipate, perceive, interpret, and respond to experiences. The events at the restaurant became the arena to replay these holograms. However, it is also a potential opportunity for changing and healing them. Perhaps, with new experiences which disconfirm old assumptions, Trina and Abby will learn to override their previous perceptions of each other.

Overview of book content

Holographic Reprocessing for Healing Trauma, Abuse, and Maltreatment is a treatment guide to help people identify their emotional and interpersonal patterns, shift their understanding and meaning of events in their lives, and engage in experiential healing (e.g., resolution, reassurance, or comfort). This is based on the concept that people form holographic memories from their experiences. Holographic reprocessing is intended for those who have experienced an interpersonal trauma (including emotional, physical abuse, harassment, maltreatment, and/or sexual trauma) or other significant trauma (such as participating, witnessing, or experiencing events during combat, a medical trauma, near-death experiences, or traumatic loss of life). This can include experiencing moral injury, self-blame, and/or complicated grief. Significant experiences such as a life trauma can leave deep impressions on people's psyches. As a result, people are motivated to enact strategies to protect and defend against further trauma. Based on these experiences, they form an experiential hologram. This refers to a theme that re-emerges throughout a person's life, including a core issue, beliefs, emotions, and coping strategies. Holographic reprocessing has a particular focus on interpersonal holograms formed from how people have been treated by other people. This overlaps with attachment theory (see Wallin, 2007) to some degree, but further delineates types of interpersonal dynamics, and these may be acquired at any time in life, not limited to early childhood.

Experiential holograms exist largely outside of conscious awareness and yet have a pervasive and profound influence on how people anticipate, perceive, interpret, and respond to life experiences. Trauma in this context is not limited to events that meet criteria for a diagnosis of posttraumatic stress (PTSD: APA 2013). In fact, holographic reprocessing is not geared specifically to treat a single diagnosis; but rather it is an approach to viewing the tailored impact of trauma—transdiagnostic. It can help mitigate symptoms related to several diagnoses such as (but not limited to) anxiety, depression and PTSD, as well as symptoms of unresolved grief, guilt, anger, and self-blame.

Holographic Reprocessing for Healing Trauma, Abuse, and Maltreatment is divided into three parts: foundation for holographic reprocessing, implementing holographic reprocessing, and status in the field. This chapter is the introduction and overview of the treatment. The second chapter discusses theoretical underpinnings, specifically, cognitive-experiential theory and attachment theory. This lays a foundation for understanding the conceptualization of the treatment. Chapter 3 delves into the foundation for how emotional memory is organized, and Chapter 4 discusses the concepts of holograms and experiential holograms.

The second part presents strategies and techniques for practical application of the treatment. Chapter 5 discusses setting the rationale and therapeutic goals for engaging in the treatment. Chapter 6 covers emotion regulation and specific skills that can be taught to clients. Strategies are offered for calming, focusing, soothing, and assisting reflection, contemplation, and awareness. These can be used in response to emotional distress, or practiced on a regular basis to reset one's resting baseline to improve emotional resilience.

Chapter 7 covers experiential discovery, how to facilitate experiential awareness, and identify patterns. Identifying patterns consists of examining one's life, including adult and childhood relationships, as an observer. What happened that caused enduring distress, persistent symptoms, or repeated re-enactments of a theme? What is the formative issue, image, belief that sustains and perpetuates itself? These patterns are discussed as *experiential holograms*. Chapter 8 presents interpersonal experiential holograms and the six components of these types of patterns. It includes exercises for self-inquiry to help clients identify their own hologram and map the components in their interpersonal relationships. More specifically, they can identify core violations (e.g, neglected, rejected, betrayed, endangered), beliefs about the self (e.g., "I'm not good enough"), and strategies used to compensate or avoid uncomfortable feelings (e.g., trying to be perfect). Chapter 9 discusses other types of experiential holograms and their core issues including responses to life threatening trauma, moral injury, and complicated grief.

Up until this part of the treatment, the focus has been on identifying issues and affect regulation. Chapter 10 is where the treatment shifts to a focus on change factors. The first factor is considering context as a new way to perceive the past. It provides various strategies to facilitate reappraisal and holistic restructuring. In spite of leading to real self-reinforcing consequences, the essence of a pattern is called into question by broadening one's perspective to consider context. Several strategies are discussed. A metaphor is offered to facilitate the observer vantage point of viewing one's life from the perspective of an observing eagle. This is in contrast to the field vantage point where one is in the event, on the ground in the field as a field mouse. The observer vantage point facilitates considering the agendas of other people or circumstances. Various strategies are offered such as *multiple truths, age comparison, hindsight advantage,* and *putting blame where blame is due (e.g., it takes a thief, and poetic justice)*, to reach a new understanding, cognitive shifts, and alterations in meaning. Other strategies may include considering a *meta-reframe* that provides a broad inclusive explanation.

The second change factor is releasing through imagery. This may include *imagery reprocessing*. Chapter 11 provides practical steps for imagery reprocessing, an imagery-based procedure where clients imagine visiting their younger self. Clients first write a letter to their younger self, then utilizing the observer vantage point, they approach the scene using guided imagery. Once in the scene, clients imagine visiting their younger self. They are asked, "What would you like to say?" "What would you like to do?" with the intention to offer a message of healing (e.g., "It was not your fault," "I will take care of you from now on.") (see Katz, 2005). Several case examples will be used throughout the text.

Chapter 12 focuses on post-treatment integration and follow-up support. Once the hologram has been reprocessed, clients may need to work on additional skills, set goals, and make a life plan. It also discusses booster reprocessing, and changing one's attitude from a defensive stance to embracing opportunities to fully engage in life.

Chapters 13 and 14 constitute the third part on status in the field. This includes a comparison of holographic reprocessing with other trauma treatments to delineate unique contributions of this treatment approach. Current outcome research is summarized in the final chapter demonstrating a growing empirical evidence base.

Holographic reprocessing is a cognitive-experiential approach

Holographic reprocessing is grounded in Epstein's Cognitive Experiential theory (CET: Epstein, 2014; Epstein & Epstein, 2016). CET proposes that we have two systems for processing information: the rational (cognitive) and the experiential (emotional) systems (Table 1.1). The rational system processes facts, theories, and abstract thoughts using logic and analytical thinking. It is slow to consider data, but quick to change. In contrast, the experiential system processes information quickly and in spite of new data,

Table 1.1 Cognitive (rational) and experiential (emotional) systems

Cognitive (rational) system	*Experiential (emotional) system*
Conscious	Largely preconscious/implicit
Analytic	Holistic
Intentional	Automatic
Logical (reason oriented)	Emotional (sensation oriented)
Linear (cause and effect) & sequential (A + B = C)	Associations (guided by patterns, memories) (one thought associates to another)
Outcome oriented	Process oriented
Slow processing/delayed action	Fast processing/immediate action
Easily changes with new input (disconfirming data influences a change of conclusion)	Resistant to change (even with disconfirming evidence, could still feel skeptical)
Requires justification, logic, evidence, reasoning (the logic makes this true)	Self-evidently valid (I feel this so it is true)

is slow to change. It is essential for its ability to effortlessly, rapidly, and efficiently direct everyday behavior. The experiential system processes emotions, imagery, and associations.

Holographic reprocessing based on CET is both cognitive and experiential and can be flexibly applied for conceptualizing formation and resolution of symptoms. Holographic reprocessing is an integrative model examining dynamics of interpersonal relationships and root causes of symptoms while effecting change through cognitive reappraisals and learning through experiential exercises.

Comparison to major psychotherapy theories

The most influential theories in the field of psychotherapy are psychodynamic and cognitive-behavioral theories. In many ways, these theories approach conceptualization and treatment from opposite viewpoints (Table 1.2). For example, psychodynamic theory focuses on bringing forth unconscious associations from early childhood events and cognitive-behavioral theory focuses on changing learning through confronting maladaptive thinking or behaviors in the here and now. CET offers a unique approach by providing a global unified theoretical framework to explain both major schools of psychotherapy (see Epstein, 2014).

Psychodynamic theory

Psychodynamic theory proposes that people are motivated or driven by a robust unconscious that is formed from early childhood experiences. The unconscious is outside of one's awareness but is the basis for personality and interpersonal relationships. Many theorists have contributed to a large body of literature explaining the idea that there is an unconscious system influencing the conscious mind. Similarly, in CET, the experiential system is a more robust predictor of behavior than the conscious mind.

More recent theories focus on the dynamics of interpersonal relationships. Object relations, for example, proposes that early childhood relationships, particularly with parents, set expectations for future relationships. These become encoded into a person's unconscious and become the basis for re-enactments or replication of similar types of relationships. The dynamics that are learned in childhood are familiar and people consciously and unconsciously seek or are attracted to those that they find familiar, and thus, set up the likelihood for replications.

Previous experiences, particularly, those from early childhood, become a filter for expectations in new relationships. When someone projects their assumptions onto someone else, it is called transference. The response someone else has to the transference put upon them is called countertransference. Object relations theory addresses the transference and countertransference as it is expressed and acted out with the therapist in therapy.

Cognitive-behavioral theory

Cognitive-behavioral therapy (CBT) focuses on behaviors and thoughts. The behavioral component is based on behaviorism which focuses on learning models such as classical conditioning, operant learning, and social learning theories. People are viewed as the product of learning through reinforcement to strengthen the learning. Positive or negative experiences strengthen the association between objects or stimuli and experiences. For example, at the time of a car accident, a certain song playing on the radio could become associated with fear experienced at the time of the event. The song becomes a conditioned stimuli as it is associated or paired with fear. The action of change is to create new learning that overrides the old one.

Cognitive theory focuses on the interactions of thoughts, feelings, and behaviors, but mostly from the perspective that thoughts lead to emotions, and emotions lead to behaviors. From this perspective, negative thoughts described as faulty thinking (illogical, distorted, or maladaptive thinking) are the source of psychological distress. Identifying and confronting automatic faulty thinking and beliefs will improve the way a client feels and behaves. These problematic thinking styles may include all-or-nothing thinking, jumping to conclusions, overgeneralizing, mind reading, and catastrophizing, personalizing, and magnification or minimization.

Table 1.2 A comparison of major psychotherapy theories

	Psychodynamic	Holographic reprocessing (cognitive -experiential)	Cognitive-behavioral
Assumptions about the nature of people	People have impulses (biological) that need to be controlled, sublimated, and redirected. They seek pleasure and avoid pain	People have various basic needs/desires (i.e., safety, health, pleasure, self-esteem, achievement, to be loved and share a connection with others). They seek what is consistent with their needs and values	People are products of their learning/ conditioning. They learn, adapt, accommodate and assimilate information. They seek to be rational and symptom-free
Assumptions about the nature of symptoms	Symptoms result from emotional repression that need cathartic release	Symptoms are clues about one's coping responses based on past experiences resulting in cognitive and emotional patterns to protect oneself	Symptoms are an indication of a cognitive distortion and/or irrational belief. Symptoms are a result of learning
Addressing symptoms	Therapy explores origins of symptoms and defenses through associations. Insight regarding why symptoms developed should be curative	Therapy explores current and origins of symptoms via associations, and techniques to consider context for reappraisal, and engage the experiential system for an emotionally corrective experience (new learning)	Therapy explores current distortions in thoughts and beliefs, and uses cognitive techniques to confront and correct these distortions. Behavioral exposure is used for new learning which may include desensitization
Theoretical vs. technical	Therapy is theory-based and practiced as an art form of associations and discovery	Therapy is theory-based and practiced as both an art and science, discovery plus the use of cognitive and experiential techniques	Therapy is practiced as a science of specific measurable cognitive techniques
Role of emotions	Therapy uses emotions to reveal associations to underlying psycho-dynamics. Emotional release is considered cathartic and healing	Therapy uses emotions to reveal associations to underlying dynamics of the experiential system. Emotional release in and of itself is not enough to change patterns	Therapy minimizes emotional experience. Instead, the focus is to determine what thoughts generated the emotion and what behaviors are learned

	Psychodynamic	Holographic repro-cessing (cognitive-experiential)	Cognitive-behavioral
Focus in time of intervention	Origin of problem	Any time, since access to all experi-ence is available in the present	Here and now
Mode of conversation	Experiential (associations)	Experiential (associa-tions, affect, sensa-tions, imagination, metaphor, stories) and cognitive con-sidering various points of view	Intellectual (use of logic and search-ing for evidence). Use of behavioral learning schedules

Cognitive-experiential theory

CET creates a theoretical bridge to explain the major schools of psy-chotherapy by providing a global theory where two seemingly disparate approaches can find common ground (Epstein, 2012, 2014). CET is a global theory of personality that integrates significant aspects of learning theory, cognitive theory, and psychoanalytic theory. It assumes that everyone auto-matically constructs an implicit theory of reality in the course of living including theories about the self, and others, and beliefs regarding their interactions (Epstein, 2012). People's implicit theories of reality auto-matically and effortlessly direct people's everyday behavior and also influ-ence their interpretation of events, feelings, and conscious thinking. Thus, people's implicit theories of reality determine in large measure their perfor-mance and the quality of their lives.

CET is similar to a psychodynamic model where most information proces-sing is assumed to occur outside of conscious awareness, not because of repression as Freud believed, but because it is a more efficient, less effortful way of processing information in everyday life than by conscious reasoning (Epstein, 2012). CET is also similar to cognitive science in its views on how implicit beliefs are encoded, stored and retrieved. CET differs from cognitive theory by its much greater emphasis on the importance of emotions, psycho-dynamics, self/phenomenological concepts, and learning theory (Epstein, 2012).

Affect and emotion is considered to be a significant aspect of associative net-works in the experiential system. According to CET, they are particularly important in the acquisition of implicit beliefs and formation of neural networks in the experiential system. Epstein (2012) states emotions are important as they provide "a royal road to the identification of the schemas in people's implicit theories of reality." Or as the author says, "emotions are the super-highway to the experiential mind." Both highlighting that emotions are an efficient direct route to the experiential system and one's implicit theories or experiential holograms.

Chapter summary

This chapter introduces the content of holographic reprocessing. It presents Epstein's cognitive-experiential theory which delineates two systems for processing information.

Chapter 2

Theoretical foundation

This chapter presents Epstein's theory of cognitive experiential theory in more detail. Cognitive-experiential theory establishes that we have two systems for processing information: cognitive (rational) and experiential (emotional). Although people generally think of themselves as rational, we are all highly susceptible to the influence of our emotions and associations from past experiences of the experiential system. This chapter also describes attachment theory and how it relates to holographic reprocessing treatment. Attachment is the quality of internalized connection to others, also known as internal working models of relationships These theories form the theoretical foundation for holographic reprocessing. Holographic reprocessing refines attachment styles (secure vs insecure) into specific individualized working models that reside in the experiential system, which are implicit and automatic, and influence daily life. In this paradigm, the internal working model and theme of re-enactments that stem from the model are termed experiential holograms (Katz, 2005).

Case example: The fair-weather friend

Faith, came to session in a rush, apologizing for having missed last session because she had "just cut off everyone in her life." She assured me that it was nothing personal and she just cut off *everyone*. She stated she has been isolating and doesn't need people in her life "who get her down." I was curious about what happened that made her feel so hurt and vulnerable. She went on to describe how she has been "avoiding the world" by staying in her apartment with the blinds closed.

Faith is an African-American woman in her forties who is in her last year of studies in a Ph.D. program in clinical psychology. She is emotionally expressive and has a nervously excited quality to her speech. However, she tends to discount her feelings and even questions her perception of reality. She may start her sentences with, "I know this sounds crazy…" or "this is really stupid…" and end with "does that sound crazy to you?" or "you must think I am totally psycho." Although I have on occasion pointed out her

DOI: 10.4324/9781003223429-3

language, it appears to be defensive and usually with the intention of seeking reassurance.

I asked what happened that was particularly upsetting to her in the last couple of weeks. She told me how she finally got her car back from her ex-husband after he got into a crash and how she has been driving her daughter crazy with her neediness. Then she mentioned that she does not want to go to a workshop because she is avoiding her friend.

"What happened with your friend?" I asked. She described how she doesn't need a friend that will drop her at the sight of a man. She said she was fed up with feeling like left-overs and she doesn't want to be a friend of convenience. Only a few weeks ago her friend gave her a card that said, "friends forever" but now she feels that this was phony and she was forgotten as soon as her friend started dating a man.

I asked her how she felt when her friend was unavailable. She stated she felt angry and hurt and that she doesn't need friends like her in her life. I asked again what she felt. She said, "lonely, abandoned, and disappointed." I asked about her expectations in a friendship. She described how she strives to create a balance between her friends and family. Sometimes she would leave her boyfriend or husband at home to go out with her friends. She stated I don't think I am wrong for wanting a friend that doesn't disappear as soon as she gets a man in her life!

We went back to the feeling of being abandoned. She discussed her abandonment from childhood. As a newborn, she was taken away from her biological mother and adopted by a married couple. However, shortly after her arrival to her new home, her adopted mother had a psychotic break and had to be hospitalized. As an infant, this client was bounced from baby-sitter to baby-sitter. She also reported being horribly abused physically, sexually, and emotionally by both adoptive parents. As a child, going into her closet was her safest and most comforting place. I thought about her as an adult locking herself up in her dark apartment to seek safety and comfort.

She stated that she feared if her friend disappeared then so did she. She described herself as floating into nothingness. I stated that it sounded like she worried that if she doesn't hear from her friend then she ceases to exist in her friend's mind. She became tearful. We likened her feelings to a modified version of the riddle, "if a tree falls in the forest and nobody is there to hear it, does it really exist?" She stated that without acknowledgment or reassurance, she feels like she floats away into an abyss, a big, black hole of nothingness.

Her experiential hologram is about how she was ignored and left to wonder if she did indeed exist. She was literally "left in the wind" and abandoned by both her biological and adopted mothers. She also literally floated into nothingness as she dissociated during her abuse. As she got older, her addictions to alcohol, drugs, sex, rage, cigarettes, caffeine etc., kept her "floating" so she would not have to feel her pain. She learned that being present in the world was not safe.

We spent several sessions talking about getting grounded and staying present. She made great strides in these areas. But today's session was about her abandonment hologram and insecure attachment. Of the people in her life, she sought this friend as a reliable and steady companion. At least this friend could accept her the way she is now, without judging her past behaviors. But this friend fell short of being reliable and steady. It became evident that her friend's unavailability activated a very painful and deep experiential hologram for this client. It appears that she is still hoping to have adequate mirroring that she missed as an infant. She is still looking for something outside of herself to validate her existence. She feared that if she was "out of sight she would be out of mind."

I asked if she thought I was able to hold her from week to week. She looked doubtful. Then I asked her if she thinks about her clients (which I knew that she did.) She laughed and said, "Okay, you got me there."

Cognitive-experiential theory (CET)

In this case example, Faith is intelligent, thoughtful, and psychologically aware; in fact, she was a therapist herself. Rationally, she knows she exists, and yet emotionally, she was deeply triggered by the experience she had with her friend. This can be explained by the dual system of processing of the cognitive (rational) and experiential (emotional) systems described by CET. Epstein and Meier (1989) found that intelligent people do not necessarily lead healthier, happier, or more productive lives. Intelligence quotient, or IQ, was the only measure that did not correlate with measures of success in living. Instead, it was a measure of the experiential mind, the *Constructive Thinking Inventory* (CTI), that best predicted outcomes of success. Similarly in a laboratory stress test, Katz and Epstein (1991) found that students who scored low on the CTI had a longer recovery period after the stress, and more negative thoughts such as worries about being judged, and perceptions of failure. Not surprising, in another study, those with higher CTI scores were found to be able to carry higher levels of productive load (e.g., in addition to taking classes, engaging in extracurricular activities, and/or leadership responsibilities) with fewer symptoms than those who scored lower on the CTI (Epstein & Katz, 1992). These studies support the idea that emotional resilience, not IQ, is a strong predictor of outcomes of success in living.

Despite remarkable intelligence, people often do poorly in solving relationship problems, which fall primarily in the domain of the experiential system, as experiential processing biases rational processing. Epstein (2014) stated that thinking in an intense emotional state fosters gross overgeneralization, holistic rather than analytical processing, wish-fulfillment rather than realistic thinking, all-or-none categorical thinking, concrete thinking, and personalized thinking. This thinking may be considered illogical from the rational perspective but a natural by-product of emotional thinking, and are common expressions of the experiential system, even for highly intelligent people. Although emotions are often the source of irrational thinking due to their biasing influence on rational processing, they also serve a critically important function regarding implicit theories of reality in the experiential system.

In the laboratory study mentioned above, even when there was no difference in performance on the tasks, one student reported feeling stupid and focused on perceived failure, while another was able to feel good about participating in the study. It was not the task, but rather the participants' implicit theories and assumptions that influenced their interpretation of their experience. Thus, people's implicit theories of reality determine in large measure people's ability to engage in activities, manage stress, and lead quality and productive lives.

People's implicit theories of reality automatically and effortlessly direct people's everyday behavior and influences their interpretation of events, feelings, and conscious thinking. The case example of Faith demonstrates how she is operating from a theory of abandonment. This is emotionally activating which means her thinking will automatically foster gross over-generalization and other emotional thinking types of logic-distortions. While a rational conversation may seem helpful on the surface, it will likely not lead to lasting change.

Which system is best?

Both systems have strengths and weaknesses. The experiential system can quickly and efficiently process information. It is primarily influenced by emotion and, as a result, it can be impulsive and poor at dealing with abstract concepts. The rational system directs behavior through logical principles. Therefore, it is well-equipped to correct the experiential system. However, the rational system processes information slowly, and it requires a large expenditure of cognitive resources. While, the two systems are largely independent, they work best in tandem.

Imagine you are buying a car. You have your heart set on one car, but you read reports that another car is safer, has better gas mileage, and is considerably less expensive. Which one are you going to choose? Your rational mind may consider the facts, while your experiential mind considers how you will feel in your new car. You test drive the highly recommended car and it doesn't feel particularly safe when you drive it. So, you test drive the other car and it feels great and much superior to the other drive. Now, the information from the two systems may be in conflict with each other. Do you buy the highly rated one or the one that feels great? Epstein's research describes that while we would like to think we make decisions with our rational mind, when it comes to the actual decision, the experiential mind often wins out.

In order to resolve the conflict of the two systems, people use emotional reasoning such as justification (coming up with an acceptable reason), focusing on supportive or confirming evidence, ignoring disconfirming evidence, and expanding upon perceived or wishful evidence. Even if the reasoning is not fully logical, sufficient reasoning and in some cases, any reasoning, seems to satisfy both systems allowing for emotionally-driven action.

In a series of studies examining choice, participants were able to state that there is no difference in the probability of choosing a red jelly bean from two jars, both with a ratio of 1 to 10. In one jar there was one red jelly bean and nine white ones, and in the other jar there were ten red jelly beans and 90 white ones. However, when given a chance to win a cash prize, most people picked the larger jar with ten red jelly beans. When queried why this jar was chosen, participants stated they felt they had a better chance of winning, in spite of knowing the probabilities are the same! Furthermore, when one of the red jelly beans was removed from the larger jar, people still chose from it even with logical knowledge that it was less optimal (Kirkpatrick & Epstein, 1992).

Global attribution bias

Another example of how the experiential mind overrides our logic is the case of global attribution bias. To demonstrate this, undergraduate students were told a scenario where if three friends each tossed a coin and they each got a head, then they would each win $100. The first friend tossed a head. The second friend tossed a head. But the third friend tossed a tail. The third friend felt bad for letting down his friends. He blamed himself and apologized. The friends were disappointed and blamed their friend for ruining their chance to win the money. Everyone blamed the third friend and attributed the poor outcome to him, even though everyone knew a coin toss is a random event. The research used this scenario and asked students if they would take the third friend with them to Las Vegas. The majority of undergraduate students did not want to take him because they said he was "bad luck."

Not only does this study reveal that when it came to something that evoked emotion (e.g., the chance to win money), logic was abandoned. Emotional thinking distorted student's decision making. The poor outcome of a random coin toss became the basis for a global attribution that *he* was bad luck, and therefore, people felt it was prudent to ostracize him.

Similarly, victims of abuse almost invariably blame themselves and think about ways they could have or should have prevented it (of course, lacking context about the perpetrator's agenda) and in addition, others may also blame the victim. They attribute the bad outcome to the person it happened to and in so doing, distance themselves from danger. This could preserve a belief in invulnerability (e.g., "It happened to them because of them; therefore, it won't happen to me"), but it also fosters stereotypes and prejudice, and blames people who are already suffering from trauma.

Emotional thinking is categorical (all or nothing), automatic, fast, and wired for self-preservation. It is striking how quickly people turned against the third friend. Unfortunately, this demonstrates how easily people can be manipulated through their emotions, even intelligent, rational people.

Heuristics and biases

Understanding cognitive experiential theory reveals how implicit bias, and heuristics (or cognitive shortcuts) influence people's thoughts and actions. Heuristics aid mental efficiency. Can you imagine how exhausting it would be to labor over every single decision? Imagine the time and effort it would take making choices in a grocery store, ordering something for lunch, or trying to have a conversation with someone if you had to think about every word or sentence. Instead, our automatic mind effortlessly guides us through everyday life. Kahneman and Tversky have studied and documented several cognitive heuristics and ways our thinking is biased (Kahneman et al., 1982). For example, the heuristic of availability is the shortcut of easily bringing an image to mind. For example, after the release of the movie *Jaws* (Spielberg, 1975), it was noted that significantly more people avoided swimming in the ocean. It's not that the ocean changed, but images of scary deadly sharks attacking people were more prevalent in people's minds. People became irrationally afraid of sharks and deaf to alternative scientific narratives (Neff, 2015). This negative image persists almost 50 years later. Another heuristic is familiarity, where people tend to favor people, things, or places that are familiar, even if a new option is better. Given this heuristic, seeing the same product advertised repeatedly, or the same political candidate on the front-page news repeatedly increases the likelihood to purchase or vote for that which is familiar. People are also influenced by their mood, known as the affect heuristic, where they perceive a decision as having more benefits and lower risks when they are in a positive mood, and the same decision viewed as having less benefits and more potential negative risks when they are in a negative mood.

Strong emotions, especially ones like fear, anger, and hate hijack rational thinking and activate the primitive fight/flight/freeze system of the autonomic nervous system (discussed in more detail in Chapter 6). This biological system is designed to mobilize against threat and danger. In addition, the experiential system processes associations where certain words, labels, stereotypes can be linked to images and emotions. Those words become conditioned to induce an automatic feeling. For example, if people who were avid supporters of opposite political parties were thrown into a conversation, it could likely arouse a host of emotions, potentially leading to arguments, name calling, and stereotypes. Strong emotions would interfere with an ability to have a rational discourse, cooperation, or shared problem solving. Categorical thinking such as right versus wrong, all or nothing, us versus them, good versus bad is experiential thinking. On the other hand, heightening categorical thinking, increases polarity and has the benefit of strengthening in-group loyalty. If someone really wants to win followers, then it behooves them to fan the flames of emotion, the stronger the better, the more outrageous the better, the more threatening the better, to cultivate in-group loyalty. In particular, fear and hate activate a deep survival response. These emotions cause dysregulation of the nervous system, a release of a host of neurochemical responses, heightened memory of feared stimuli, and thus, effectively disengages rational thought.

Nonetheless, even when people can calmly access their logic, knowledge in and of itself, does not necessarily predict behavior. For example, people may say they know they should do a behavior and yet they do not. There are many examples: from wanting to engage in exercise, changing one's diet, breaking-up from an unhealthy romantic relationship, changing a boring job, confronting a family member, stop smoking, etc. where people say they want to change but they don't. Something else is guiding their decisions—in their experiential mind. Their experiential mind may be responding to a feeling, image, or memory, perhaps an uncomfortable or painful experience from the past or anticipation of an uncomfortable or painful experience in the future. Why would they want to change if they are anticipating some form of discomfort? Again, this is largely outside of one's awareness, they may not know why, but they "just don't feel like changing." It is the experiential system that blocks as well as supports behavior change.

The experiential system is slow to change even when presented with facts or new information. If someone, for example, was attacked in an elevator, logic alone may be insufficient for change. A therapist can confront distortions in logic, and present data that elevators are no more or less dangerous than stairs. The client nods in agreement and states that it "makes sense." However, the client leaves the office, walks to the elevator, and experiences heart palpitations, shortness of breath, an intense wave of fear, and then decides to take the stairs. What happened? The therapist presented a solid case of logic, but the client's experiential system took over. The elevator triggered threatening images and intrusive thoughts about the attack. Of course, the client would want to avoid danger and seek safety.

The experiential system processes information quickly and is largely outside of conscious awareness. For example, imagine someone is walking in a park and glances to one side to see a tree that looks like it is ready to fall. Using the cognitive-rational system, the trajectory of the tree could be estimated, and calculations suggest that it would likely fall their way. This would be inefficient and dangerous. Luckily, using the experiential system, the person is able to glance towards the tree, activating the automatic bio-logical alarm system to run. Once out of danger, the experience is processed in the rational system. The person, out of breath from running, realizes, "Wow, I could have been hit by that tree!" The experiential system is fast and the rational system is slow.

On the other hand, the rational system processes information slowly. It is in a position to correct the emotionally-driven automatic response of the experiential system. It is this ability that allows us to consciously control our automatic responses and have capabilities such as affect regulation and behavior change. Cognitive therapy helps people confront the distortions of emotional thinking.

Thus, the two systems have equally important advantages and dis-advantages. The rational system provides the advantage of solving problems, processing factual information, drawing inferences, and has the power to correct, modulate, and override emotional thinking with conscious thought, cognitive restructuring, and practice. The experiential system has the advantage of effortlessly directing everyday behavior. It also has the advan-tage of promoting empathy, interpersonal connection, humor, creativity, and intuition, and protecting oneself from potential danger. Neither is superior, but rather they are complementary, and both provide different adaptive ways of processing information (Epstein, 2014).

In holographic reprocessing, the knowledge of these two systems is used to help access, identify, and understand persistent patterns and symptoms. Several strategies are used to help people become aware that they are living in a pattern. They learn about their life themes growing from formative experiences, and this provides a logic to their behavior, choices, and reac-tions. However, the goal for treatment is change. Epstein proposed that the experiential system must be activated in order to generate permanent emo-tional change, achieved by communicating with the experiential system in its own medium. The experiential system communicates through emotions, imagery, story, and metaphor. New learning such as through an actual new experience or evoking emotional learning through vicarious experiences, or imagined experiences can lead to change (Epstein, 2014). An emotionally corrective learning experience disconfirms old patterns, and sets new ones in place. Change has to be felt. Even if the change involves a new perception or insight, the change still needs to connect emotionally. This could be releas-ing negative emotions such as blame, fear, and guilt, or activating positive ones such as comfort, safety, forgiveness, and compassion.

Therapeutic change happens through emotionally corrective experiences.

Metaphors, insight, and imagery to reach the experiential system

Epstein (2014) discusses that metaphors provide a link between the two processing systems. Although presented in words, they engage the experi-ential system by evoking images, associations, and emotions that make the information they present more engaging and comprehensible than the same information presented in prose (e.g., Ralph is really angry, vs Ralph is like a raging lion).

He also stated that "insight occurs when a person has a new and correct understanding in the rational system in a manner that reaches and corrects an invalid belief in the experiential system" (personal communication with Dr Epstein, 2013). While insight is cognitive, it can reach and correct the experiential system for lasting change.

Another cognitive strategy to reach the experiential system is imagery. Imagery is particularly powerful in reaching the experiential system. Imagining an experience can have cognitive and behavioral effects similar to experience itself (Epstein & Pacini, 2001). Holographic reprocessing uses all three of these cognitive strategies, metaphors, insight, and imagery, to effect change in the experiential system.

Ways to effect change in the experiential system:

1   In vivo or actual lived experiences (engaging in new behaviors)
2   Fantasy, metaphor, stories (evoking emotional images using imagination)
3   Vicarious experience (imaging what it would feel like)
4   Emotional activation (building new associations)
5   Physical/sensory activation (building new associations)

Attachment theory

As the work of Harry Harlow (Halow & Harlow, 1962) found, newborn monkeys have a biological need for nurturing touch and seeking the proximity of an adult monkey for safety and soothing. Infant rhesus monkeys were separated from their mothers at six to twelve hours after birth. Even when a wire mother was the source of nourishment, the infant monkey spent a greater amount of time clinging to a cloth surrogate. Harlow's monkeys showed that seeking a relationship with a mother was independent of feeding needs.

These observations were the foundation of *attachment theory* (see Ainsworth, 1969; Bowlby, 1969, 1973; Main & Solomon, 1986). Attachment or connection to one's mother or other caregiver provides a safe haven or feeling of security for a child. A secure relationship fosters healthy exploration of the world because the child knows he or she can come back to the caregiver for safety. When the child becomes upset, the caregiver soothes the child and thereby, teaches the child how to self-soothe. The child learns, "I'm okay." Modern day attachment theory can be understood as a theory of regulation (Schore & Schore, 2008) starting with the relationship between infant and caregiver, and then is replicated in adult romantic relationships (Hazan & Shaver, 1987).

Securely attached babies/children are able to explore their environment when they feel safe and seek solace when they do not.

John Bowlby theorized that from early infancy people develop an inner-working model of attachment that enables them to recognize patterns of interactions not only with a caregiver, but these patterns then generalize to others. The inner-working model influences a general expectation of how others will act, and thus, also influences the individual's behavior (see Wallin, 2007, for more information about attachment theory). The primary caregiver must be "good enough" for the child to feel safe enough and develop an inner-working model of trust and safety. If the caregiver is unreliable, this leaves the child feeling insecure.

Insecure attachment can interfere with neuro-biological and physical development, self-esteem, and social functioning. As Braun and Bock (2011) outline, the maturation of critical brain development depends on experience. Based on an infant's emotional experiences, especially with the primary caregiver, the infant's brain will develop, organize, and learn. Exposure to an enriched environment with adequate stimulation, attentive care, and loving comfort, facilitates healthy development. Conversely, if the infant is raised in a deprived environment, or experiences trauma during early childhood, it may leave scars in prefrontal-limbic function, brain regions that are essential for emotional behavior, learning, and memory (Braun & Bock, 2011).

Formation of a secure attachment

Attachment develops from birth and depends on the quality of the relationship with a primary caregiver. Attachment continues to develop, particularly through the early years when young children begin to explore their new and exciting world. If there is a potential danger, the caregiver is there to hold boundaries. If the child confronts something scary or threatening, they can come back to the caregiver for comfort. The caregiver is the safe haven to calm and soothe the child. The caregiver lovingly says, "it's ok," and the child internalizes the soothing.

Secure attachment is a combination of four elements: feeling loved enough, safe enough, trusting that a caregiver will hold boundaries and rules for protection, and having enough freedom and trust in oneself and the world to go out and explore—knowing there is a safety net of a caregiver ready to protect and provide comfort (Figure 2.1).

In holographic reprocessing, if one or more of these elements is not sufficient, then it may impact the person's ability to function and form relationships. For example, for people who did not feel loved enough but had no threat of safety, they may feel emptiness inside and a disconnection from others. If this is coupled with overly-permissive parents (e.g., not paying attention or not providing guidance, rules, or limits), they may feel neglected. If on the other hand, parents were strict and critical, and constricted

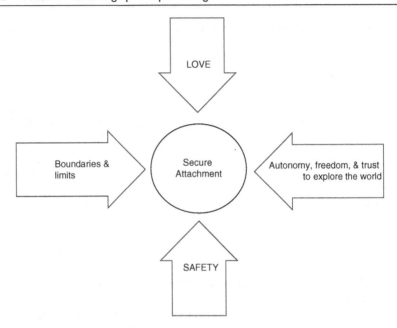

Figure 2.1 Elements for a secure attachment.

their children's ability to take the initiative or make decisions, they may suffer from feeling rejected and not good enough.

If children feel unsafe growing up due to a threatening environment, or caregivers were unpredictable, threatening, or abusive—then they may feel anxious inside. If this is coupled with permissive parents or those with no respect for rules, agreements, or boundaries, they may experience feeling betrayed. If feeling unsafe was coupled with strict, constrictive, or overly critical parents, they may feel a constant threat or endangerment.

Impact of secure and insecure attachment

Those with secure attachment have greater self-esteem, emotional health, positive affect, initiative, social competence, and better concentration. Not surprisingly, attachment is a robust predictor of success in living. It is associated with a higher global measure of overall functioning and decreased symptoms (Muller & Rosenkranz, 2009). Secure attachment may also have a protective factor as those with a secure attachment had fewer PTSD symptoms three months following a traumatic event, and a decreased reliance on avoidance strategy (specifically substance use) to alleviate negative affect related to the traumatic event (Benoit et al., 2010).

In contrast, insecure attachment, such as attachment anxiety is a robust predictor of poorer outcomes and mental health problems including risk of mental illness, more physical health problems, higher divorce rates, lower financial success, more depression, shorter life expectancy and suicide (Dagan et al., 2018; Mikulincer & Shaver, 2016; Stanton & Campbell, 2014). Attachment anxiety has been associated with poorer mental health outcomes compared to secure individuals in nearly all of these studies.

Numerous studies have evidenced a link between insecure attachment and PTSD in adulthood (Declercq & Willemsen, 2006; Fraley et al., 2006; Kanninen et al., 2003; Zakin et al., 2003). A hypothesized pathway is that insecurity internalized as a negative view of self adversely impacts coping, which increases the vulnerability for the development of PTSD following a trauma later in life (Muller et al., 2000). This may also lead to increased risk of self-blame as a way to make sense of traumatic life events (Liem & Boudewyn, 1999).

In the case example at the beginning of this chapter, Faith had a deep insecurity of being left alone to such an extent that she felt she didn't exist. She did not have a solid or secure foundation; therefore, she had not internalized a sense of a stable self. Because of her lack of stable parenting from birth, therapy required a lengthier course of treatment to provide her with a secure base, to teach affect regulation skills, and help her internalize a more positive self-concept. She was seeking a positive attachment with her friend and wanted her to be a reliable, positive, loving figure, likely to address an unfulfilled wish for a stable mother that she did not have. But her wish was also likely unrealistic, as her friend may not have agreed to be her surrogate mother. This sets Faith up to continue to feel disappointed and abandoned. The attachment is the quality of her internalized connection to others. The experiential hologram is the interpersonal pattern that she is replicating.

Improved attachment post-treatment

While attachment is typically viewed as a trait (e.g., stable over time), there is a growing literature demonstrating that attachment can improve with new experiences with emotionally attuned others (e.g., a relationship or psychotherapy) (Mikulincer et al., 2013). The term earned security is used to describe the development of secure attachment later in life among individuals that were previously characterized by attachment-related insecurity. Earned security is also related to the ability to refrain from recapitulation of past negative experiences into the future (Phelps et al., 1998). Roisman et al. (2002) found that individuals who developed earned security as an adult have emotionally close and intimate relationships, akin to individuals with secure attachment without the internalized emotional distress characteristic of individuals with insecure attachment.

Holographic reprocessing proposes to target change at the experiential level leading to deep change, including internalized attachment. It seemed necessary to put this claim to the test. Sixty-two graduates of the warrior renew program completed the *Relationship Scales Questionnaire* (RSQ:

Griffin & Bartholomew, 1994) and Brief Symptom Inventory (BSI-18; Derogatis, 2000) before and after 12 weeks of group treatment (Katz et al., 2016). Results demonstrated that these treatment graduates significantly improved perceived secure attachment and reduced insecure-fearful attachment. Post-treatment RSQ scales *secure*, *fearful*, and *dismissive* scales were significantly correlated with reports of post-treatment symptoms. Specifically, *secure attachment* was inversely related to symptoms of anxiety and depression, while *fearful attachment* was related to higher scores of anxiety and depression, and *dismissive attachment* was related to higher depression.

This is particularly meaningful, given that of the 62 graduates, 61 reported more than one event of trauma across the lifespan including childhood, and military sexual trauma, and adult/domestic violence. Most experienced multiple events in more than one time frame. Thus, this adult sample of women veterans had complex, repeated sexual trauma in the context of power dynamics (e.g., childhood, military, and domestic) where they could not have easily escaped. The implication is that improving perceived attachment may facilitate change toward a more secure pattern of relating with others (Mikulincer & Shaver, 2008).

Chapter summary

1   Cognitive-experiential theory establishes that we have two systems for processing information: cognitive (rational) and experiential (emotional).
2   Although people think of themselves as rational, we are all highly susceptible to the influence of our emotions, and associations from past experiences of the experiential system.
3   We can influence, change, and learn new patterns by engaging the experiential system.
4   Attachment is the quality of internalized connection to others, also known as internal working models of relationships.
5   While much research supports childhood attachment is a robust predictor of adult outcomes, both positive and negative attachment events can change the trajectory.

   a   Negative experiences such as sexual trauma and abuse can disrupt attachment as it is trauma perpetrated by another person, and typically impacts one's social functioning.
   b   Positive healing experiences such as having a loving consistent partner, or positive therapy experience can improve attachment.

6   Holographic reprocessing defines working models that reside in the experiential system, which are implicit and automatic, and influence daily life. In this paradigm, the internal working model leads to a theme of re-enactments that stem from the model are termed *experiential holograms* (Katz, 2005).

Chapter 3

Neural networks and associative learning

This chapter discusses how memories associate for holistic processing. Neural networks develop for efficient processing of important information such as the task of detecting potential threats. They become a filter for how people anticipate, perceive, interpret, and respond to life experiences. This is explained through a metaphor of wearing virtual reality goggles.

Case example: The orphanage

A Caucasian male veteran woke up in the middle of the night because he thought he heard a noise. He went downstairs, waking up his wife and daughter. He saw them and said, "Who are you?" He didn't recognize them. He got his clothes and left the house, he said, "I am going to catch a flight to Vietnam." His son-in-law called the police. The police asked him what he was doing. The veteran said he needed a ride to the airport. He said it was 1969 and he had to get back to Vietnam. Instead, an ambulance came and took him to the Emergency Room (ER). He was referred for therapy.

In therapy, he recalled what happened that night where he ended up in the ER. He said he thought he was on leave and needed to go back to Vietnam. I asked why did he have to go back? He said there was a place he visits, an orphanage, and part of the orphanage was blown up. He wanted to go find the guy who did this.

Then he remembered that he actually did find the guy, he beat him up and believed he might have killed him, but was not sure. He walked back to the orphanage and said he would help clean it up. The sisters couldn't do it. He cleaned it up for the sisters. He never talked about it. He finished his tour of duty and went back to the states and put the event out of his mind, although he harbored a strange feeling that he didn't belong in the states. When 9/11 happened, he started crying and said he couldn't stop. He was admitted to the hospital.

DOI: 10.4324/9781003223429-4

He said he has a long history of getting treatment. He has had flash-backs on a regular basis about 1–2 times a month, sometimes more. Sometimes it's like having a seizure, he goes to the hospital and then he calms down. He said he falls asleep and finds himself in Vietnam, watching things happen. He has been having these dreams since 9/11. He is on medication which seems to help, but he still has these episodes on a regular basis.

He has had therapy for PTSD including CPT, anger management, and a class for coping skills. He said he handles it by putting memories in a box. He tells himself, "It's going to be a good day today." He tries to remember to be thankful for the good things in his life.

We outlined two different ways to move forward with this:

1   We could work on ways to stay in the present: such as smelling euca-lyptus oil to help him snap back to the present (this can be used for nightmares, triggers, flashbacks, anxiety), avoid military shows, limit exposure to the news
2   Or we could work to complete the past: addressing *why* he is stuck back in Vietnam. I introduced the idea of neural networks and how emotions connect memories. We discussed the image of a string of holiday lights where the string is an emotion and the lights are all the events that are consistent with the emotion. He was able to relate. We discussed reprocessing the networks by viewing the past in context, from his current age perspective to see the younger version of himself as a 19-year-old who had the courage to help. This process helps complete grief and addresses the underlying issue of why he keeps wanting to go back

He said he wanted to complete the past.

At the next session, we discussed the experiential vs logical part of the brain. He said in his flashbacks he needs to get to a certain place. He said, "I need to help the children." During his flashbacks, he doesn't recognize anyone. We discussed that he gets into a hypnotic trance. He said he gets upset and his mind clicks, and he thinks that he has to get a vehicle, and drive to the orphanage.

But after 9/11, he started crying. He said he couldn't stop thinking about the orphanage. He remembers the sisters told him the orphanage was bombed because of "the American." He was consumed with thoughts of what he did. He said he could see it, but couldn't change anything. "If only I could go back there and change it." "If I hadn't been introduced to the orphanage, this wouldn't have happened." He believed the orphanage was bombed because he was the American who visited them.

But as we talked, more of the context was revealed. He said the children were half Vietnamese and half American. These children were hated because they were half American. I asked if he thought the orphanage could have been bombed because the children were half American? He thought about it and said, "Yes, it probably was."

We discussed his spiritual beliefs. He said he believes souls go to heaven and God is there to take care of them. He said the body dies but the soul and spirit go to heaven.

At the next session, he said he was feeling less anxious and feeling better. I asked why he thought so. Prior to that conversation, he hadn't thought about the children being half American. This gave the event context for why they were killed.

Then we discussed what he thinks about the 19-year-old who was in Vietnam. He started talking about his childhood before he signed up for the military. When he was a child, he lived in the country side. Starting around age five, he started going to his neighbor's farm. They had beef cows and he would feed them in the morning. The farm was also a butchery. When he got a bit older, he would help clean up. He did this until he was age 15. Then he went into the service.

We discussed that his work on the farm, in a way prepared him to help clean up at the orphanage after the bombing. His childhood experiences at the farm, enabled him, trained him, prepared him for an important job that nobody else could have done. The nuns could not have done it. He helped them. He was uniquely poised to be able to help.

He said he never thought of it that way. He said maybe he was spiritually guided to help. He put his memories away for 50 years, although intrusive thoughts grabbed his attention, and nearly destroyed him. But now looking back on his life, he can see it in a new way. Looking at his life and connecting all of the dots, he thought—if he didn't have his childhood, he couldn't have done what he did in Vietnam. If he didn't join the military, he would not have met his wife.

We discussed if he could meet his younger self (at age 19 in Vietnam), what would he tell him? He told him, "It wasn't his fault." He told him, "He did a good job to help the Sisters." He said, "Even if I didn't go there, it probably would have happened anyway. They had their agenda." He was letting go of his responsibility for something that was not his.

He discussed his experience of clam digging, when his boots get stuck in mud. He described his mind had been stuck in the mud for all of these years. He said he feels the images are deep in his mind, like fire inside of him. We discussed cooling the images, putting them away, allowing them to be there but more distant. We discussed grieving the loss of the children. He used imagery of letting them go: like a bouquet of balloons, visualizing letting them float up to heaven, wishing them well.

He said he appreciated being able to talk about these things. He said the flashbacks have stopped. He hasn't had one since we started talking. He was having them once a week for a while, but they seemed to have completely stopped. He used to feel that going back to Vietnam was a purpose, but now something in him has shifted. He has other things to think about like his grandchildren.

Four months later, we spoke for a brief follow-up session. He said he has had no flashbacks since we spoke. He said he feels the past has been resolved. The images used to be in color, but now they are in black and white. He no longer interacts with the past imagery. He said, "It's gone now, it's not my responsibility. Now, it's just a memory." He was appreciative and he said he is glad it has changed. His wife got on the phone to say, "It's a miracle."

Associations and emotions in holographic reprocessing

Holographic reprocessing therapy works to identify emotional and interpersonal themes or core violations and patterns (across events over time). It uses emotions as a gateway for further inquiry and understanding by finding out why a person thinks and acts a certain way. Note this is not an intellectual conversation or something that people can readily explain, but rather the inquiry is on the emotional level, such as asking about associations, images, feelings, and memories. This is from a phenomenological perspective, viewing reality from the perspective of the viewer. The viewer reveals the personalization of the experience such as, "What does this mean to me or about me?" or in this case example, how he believed what happened in the orphanage was his fault. When people are experiencing events, they are perceiving what is happening to them. They are occupied by their experience and how to best respond in the moment. They are actively processing input from their sensory awareness. When there is trauma, they are flooded with neurobiological responses to mobilize resources to handle the emergency. Non-essential blood flow such as to the frontal lobe is decreased. The rational-cognitive thinking part of the brain is pushed to the side. Only later, retrospectively, can the person reflect about what happened. Insight occurs retrospectively.

In this case example, he held a narrative about the event that was consistent with his emotions of horror and grief. However, his narrative lacked critical information about the context. When he was able to reflect about his experience, he was able to piece it together in a new way. The bomb had shattered something inside of him, and he had left a piece of himself in the orphanage. He needed to retrieve it. Intuitively, he knew he had to go back to Vietnam, but his conscious-rational self didn't know why. When his current age self was able to reflect on his experience, he was able to see it from a new perspective and resolve his past.

Holographic reprocessing is practiced flexibly and tailored to an individual. In this case example, we did not map his pattern. For him, the issue was flashbacks to the orphanage and what happened with the bomb. I had first assumed the issue was unresolved grief which is often associated with guilt, self-blame, and shame. But what was revealed, was that he thought they were bombed because of the hatred of the American, meaning him. He personalized this event instead of seeing the context of the War. That was the piece that he needed to understand, that his core issue of self-blame was inaccurate. They didn't bomb the place because of him, they bombed it because they didn't want half American children infiltrating their culture. With this insight, he could release his self-blame, and then his grief. But the piece that was truly transformational, was seeing his unique ability to help. Not only was it not his fault, he was uniquely poised to help the nuns. This shifted his perception from being the villain to the hero. He truly was a hero who stepped up to do an unthinkable act of selfless service. He was able to appreciate the duty of his 19-year-old self. He was able to imagine visiting his 19-year-old self and deliver a message of gratitude to him.

The treatment was brief. It was conducted in six sessions over a ten-week period with a four-month follow-up session. His wife joined the last call to say thank you and confirmed his shift.

What does your future look like if you live from the past?

What happens if the past serves as one's reference point for perceptions, interpretations, and reactions? Then likely the person will continue to behave in ways that perpetuate these perceptions. While this may be efficient for quick processing, it may also be limiting. As the veteran described, his "mind was stuck in mud" keeping his thoughts focused on the past. A metaphor to explain this is driving a car while looking in the rearview mirror. If one focuses predominantly on what is in the rearview mirror, then it would be difficult to drive forward without getting into an accident. Unresolved trauma has a way of grabbing one's attention, keeping the focus on the past.

In the book, *Warrior Renew* (Katz, 2014) an exercise is offered asking people to choose a flavor of a cupcake while being completely in the present. Almost invariably, participants of the exercise make a choice but it is based on a past experience. They may say, "because I like it," or "because I've never tried that one before." Either way, the choice is based on previous experience. Choosing completely in the present usually stumps adults, as has been the case doing this exercise with over a hundred adults.

I was giving a workshop to a class of junior high school students and challenged them with this exercise. A 13-year-old boy raised his hand and said, "Oh that's easy! Eenie, meenie, minie, moe, I choose this one!" It was brilliant. He had no story, associations, explanations, justifications… he just chose. I love that story because he was such a great teacher of being present. He embraced a freedom that most adults struggle to find.

The reason most adults struggle with this simple exercise is that they have well-developed neuro-structures or networks to efficiently aid in the recall of memories. The word "pumpkin pie," or "strawberry ice-cream" evokes an image, a memory, a set of associations. Some love it, or hate it, or some may have an allergic reaction, whatever the association, the word is not neutral. The associations are automatic, influencing their thoughts, feelings, and behaviors.

Associative learning

When it comes to a trauma or an emotionally threatening event, learning is attenuated by intense emotion and neurochemical release. For example, if someone was attacked by a tiger, they will form a neural association to quickly and efficiently process any cue that could be another tiger in order to mobilize against the threat. This is adaptive learning. Maybe an efficient recognition of potential threats, will hasten one's response and avoid or prepare for the attack.

However, this person walks into a room with orange carpet and experiences a panic attack. What happened? The person may not be aware of why they are having this reaction. If you asked them, they are aware that they are standing on an orange carpet. They can tell you that yes, they are standing on a carpet, and not a tiger. So why is the body responding with such intense anxiety? This can be explained by the rational-experiential system. Logically, the person knows that they are on a carpet, but experientially, images of the trauma are activated and a host of chemical responses are released engaging the hypothalamus-pituitary-adrenal system (HPA axis) mobilizing the body's natural mechanism to run or fight.

The sight of orange carpet triggered implicit recall of past trauma. The reaction is not to the carpet, but to memories of trauma. The body does not differentiate if the origin of the message is from the current experience or a recall of a past experience. The perception of potential danger activated by implicit memory results in a cascade of neuro-chemical reactions, mobilizing the body to respond to threat or danger. Associative learning increases the probability to continue to live from the past, thereby, serving to replicate past experiences moving into the future. Furthermore, repeated experiences reinforce the learning network so that it becomes more efficient and more automatic. This is consistent with a neural network model of memory consolidation and retrieval (Recanatesi et al., 2015). However, evidence also suggests that experiences are coded holistically across the brain as holograms and can be activated and retrieved (Bryukhovetskiy, 2015). Quite possibly, there may be multiple systems of encoding, storing, and retrieving information depending on the type, quality, and function of the information or memory.

In *Warrior Renew* (Katz, 2014), an example is presented about a character named George who asked his friend Mary to go to a party. She declines, stating that she hates parties. Surprised, George asks, "Why do you hate parties so much?" She responds that they are loud, people are obnoxious, and mostly they are "just annoying." He convinces her to go to a quiet dinner party with the option to leave at any time. Reluctantly, she agrees. If she has a good experience (e.g., engages with others, laughs, enjoys the meal and conversation) her thoughts about hating parties may start to shift. She may be more open to going to another party in the future. Even if she is still a bit hesitant, the more positive experiences she has, the easier it will be for her to go to another party. Disconfirming experiences weaken the associated feeling of hating parties, and begins to build a new neural network. However, if she went to the party with George and had a bad experience, her neural network is reinforced, strengthening her belief that she hates parties. She will likely be more reluctant to go to any party. Avoidance of parties will keep her neural network intact and reinforce her belief that parties are to be hated and, therefore, should be avoided.

One way to address this issue is to encourage exposure to parties and with repeated positive experiences her negative association will be extinguished. However, this means Mary has to do the very thing she hates most, which is to go to parties. She may not agree to this. If this was part of a treatment, she could drop out of the treatment before her negative feelings resolve. She risks reinforcing her hatred of parties if she has a bad experience. Furthermore, she may approach parties in such a way that she perpetuates a negative experience, or she may be acutely sensitive to perceiving her experience as bad. In other words, she expects to hate parties, anticipates a bad outcome, is more likely to perceive and interpret experiences as bad, and then reacts in ways that confirm her belief.

However, there is another way to address this issue by delving deeper into *why* Mary feels this way. The focus shifts from behavioral exposure, to addressing the underlying cause. What happened in Mary's past that formed this strong opinion about parties? Based on the principle of association in the experiential system, the strong emotion can be used as a gateway to understanding more about why Mary hates parties. In this case, Mary was asked, "What do you think of when you think of parties?" She was instructed to take a couple of deep breaths, as relaxing facilitates access to her experiential system where implicit thinking resides. She was asked to imagine being at a party and to describe what she experienced. She said, "When I think about parties, I'm at a large party, the music is thumping, I'm in the middle of the dance floor, dancing... people closing in around me... sweating bodies. I feel trapped! I can't breathe!" She suddenly opens her eyes, catching her breath. "I know why I hate parties. It reminds me of when I was sexually assaulted, even though it happened in the back of a truck. Isn't that strange?"

Mary associated sweaty bodies, trapped, and can't breathe with her sexual assault experience. Her hatred of parties has nothing to do with parties, but rather her mind associated parties with threat and danger. With further inquiry, Mary was asked if she felt that way before. Focusing on the feeling of being trapped, she thought about growing up. Her parents argued and she hated it. She felt their yelling closing in on her. She had a distinct memory of putting a pillow over her ears to block the noise. When asked if she had other experiences of feeling trapped, she described being the go-between for two friends who would gossip about each other to her. She hated it, but didn't connect these experiences until now. Mary has a pattern, or experiential hologram of being trapped. This pattern is deeply encoded and something associated with strong emotions, that she hates.

Emotions organize memories

Emotions play a key role in the efficiency of the recall of memories. If a strong emotion is associated with an experience, then related details are more easily remembered while non-related details are obscured. For example, Albert remembers that the last holiday family gathering was horrible because he had an argument with his husband who stormed out of the house. Albert worried that his husband offended his mother and embarrassed the family. He may remember his feelings of humiliation, frustration, and loneliness. However, he may have forgotten about the tasty meal they had, or how his younger sister helped him set the table. There were, most likely, many pleasant details about the dinner that are overlooked in his narrative as they are overshadowed by the negative emotions associated with the evening. But not everyone at the dinner will recall the same details. Maybe his younger sister felt ignored and invisible as all the attention focused on Albert, as usual. Maybe his husband remembers getting some fresh air so he wouldn't say something he regretted, to protect Albert from embarrassment. People will remember details that provide confirming evidence to their existing beliefs, and disregard disconfirming evidence. Albert, his husband, and his sister will each recall details that are most salient to them, constructing a narrative of the evening and reinforcing their associations and memories.

Every day we are bombarded with a mass of stimuli, too much to possibly absorb. We clump things together, give things labels, categorize, simplify, stereotype, and use heuristics, in order to be more efficient in our processing of information. One way of organizing our vast array of experience is through our emotions. When we are experiencing a certain emotion, we can easily recall other experiences that are associated with the same emotion. This is state-dependent learning. When in a certain emotional state, information that was learned in the same emotional state will be more easily recalled. For example, people who are depressed are more likely to remember depressing experiences than non-depressed people.

When someone is grieving a loss, they are more likely to remember other losses. Emotions facilitate the retrieval of memories that are consistent with the emotion.

State-dependent learning is a fundamental concept in understanding how experiential holograms are activated. Like a string of holiday lights, as mentioned earlier, the string is a particular emotion and each light represents an event that is associated with that emotion (Figure 3.1). For example, if the string was related to feeling betrayed, and something in the present evokes the same feeling, then the string of lights would be plugged in. All the lights on the string light up. Now, the person is not only reacting to the current situation, but to all the other events that bring up the same feeling.

> Emotions organize memories. When a particular emotion is activated, memories consistent with that emotion become more easily remembered. Thus, people may be reacting to one event, but also to all past related events.

Imagine now that this string of lights is really a network of neurons. Instead of a single line of lights, imagine an intricate pattern of lights that are strung together. The network facilitates recollection of emotions, thoughts, physical sensations, and of course, visual, auditory, olfactory, and gustatory sensations. The memory is not only a verbal recounting of the event (a story), but also a three-dimensional holographic reproduction of the perception of the event. The more experiences that attach to the network, the more robust, nuanced, and efficient it can become.

While efficiency may be beneficial to protect against real threats and dangers, trauma-based networks run the risk of overfitting experiences. Overfitting means perceiving events in the present as related to one's network of perceptions even when it is not accurate. It is a highly sensitized reaction resulting in activating trauma-based reactions when there is no actual threat or danger. The response to the orange carpet example presented earlier in this chapter is an example of overfitting. A system that was designed to be productive is now counterproductive.

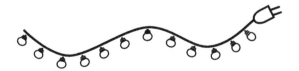

Figure 3.1 A string of holiday lights.

Addressing the blueprint, not the house

As mentioned, we tend to reference the past in the present, thereby replicating interactions consistent with the past. The past becomes part of a
network of memories that operates largely outside of our conscious awareness, in the experiential system. This network becomes our emotional-
interpersonal blueprint. It provides a template for relationships and self-
concept. The template is formed from early childhood experiences and subsequent relationships confirming beliefs and disregarding disconfirming
beliefs to develop a robust and efficient network. This is the relationship
blueprint, similar to an architectural blueprint, that is, the instructions of
how to build a house. However, what if the house built using this blueprint
has a flaw in the plumbing in the upstairs bathroom. Maybe that particular
bathroom could be fixed (or not). It becomes too problematic, so the builder
builds a new house. But the next house, built from the same blueprint, has
the same issue. In fact, all of the houses built from the same blueprint have a
similar problem.

Likewise, if the emotional-relationship blueprint has instructions that
people you love leave you, or that you will be criticized, ignored,
betrayed, or hurt, then the relationships built from this blueprint will
have these same issues. People are remarkably consistent in their relationships, creating similar dynamics. One client said, she kept dating
the same person over and over, but in a different body! In holographic
reprocessing, the focus is on changing the blueprint. The individual
houses, or relationships, can reveal what the issue is, but the treatment
is about addressing the underlying issue on the blueprint or template. If
not, the issue may persist.

A similar metaphor is that watching a movie is a projection from film. If
there is a smudge on the film, it will be present in every movie projected
from that film. The treatment addresses the film, not the projection of the
movie as it plays out on the screen.

New disconfirming experiences, effortful conscious changes, and positive
emotional experiences can help change the hologram. It is possible that new
experiences can weaken old associations, but the experiential system is slow
and resistant to change without compelling experiential evidence. It is
entirely possible, given positive influences, and concerted efforts that old
patterns can change.

Self-blame conversation

After trauma, people reflect and wonder, "Why did this happen?" And
"Why did this happen to *me*?" It is an attempt to make sense of the experience. They may review the experience, and wonder what they did, and what
they could have, or maybe should have done instead. If only they knew what

was about to happen—if only they reacted differently. They review behaviors leading up to the event, thinking that if only they didn't accept the
drink, go in the car, stay late for work, etc., then the event wouldn't have
happened. And they conclude that it is, therefore, "*my fault.*"

In my experience of treating thousands of clients with trauma, this
thought process is all too common. In fact, it is so common that it is
necessary to assess for self-blame as a critical component of healing from
trauma. Why do so many people blame themselves for an event that was
clearly the action of someone or something else?

From the vantage point of the one who was attacked, assaulted, or
abused, this narrow, emotional logic makes sense. They are viewing the
event from the perspective of what happened to them and what they
could have done to avoid or stop it. They wished it didn't happen and
regret the outcome. They might conclude that they are not good enough,
important enough, loved, safe, etc. They might conclude that they can't
trust others, or themselves, or the world is unpredictable or dangerous.
They might conclude that whatever happened is because of them,
because it happened to them. It is a closed-loop argument; while not
logical from a rational perspective, it is consistent with their experience.
Therefore, it becomes their narrative and basis for their emotional-relationship
blueprint.

Similarly, if a child experiences a trauma, or violation by a primary
caregiver, or someone important to the child, as a survival mechanism, the
child will be motivated to preserve the relationship. If the child blames
themself, then it preserves their world view that the caregiver is good and
the world is predictable. This is consistent with Janoff-Bulman's work on
people's desire for a just and predictable world (Janoff-Bulman, 1992).
From childhood to adulthood, personalization is a common (maybe automatic) reaction. People ask, "Why did this happen to me?" and they make
it personal.

The problem with this thinking is that it lacks context. When someone is
reviewing their experience as if they are still in the experience, they are only
thinking about what happened to them, and what they could have done to
prevent it. It is as if they are only seeing the event through a small peephole,
not even considering the rest of the picture. This limited perspective keeps
them stuck, re-experiencing trauma and wishing they could have stopped it.
It lacks considering a bigger understanding, the roles of all involved, their
motivation, agenda, and intention. It also lacks remembering one's own
context, what they were thinking, feeling, responding to at the time. A lack
of context leads to personalization and erroneous conclusions about the self,
others, and the world. It fuels emotional thinking, formation of trauma-
based associative networks, and beliefs designed to protect (such as avoiding
parties), but really only serve to perpetuate false beliefs that limit one's life.

Self-blame can also be a red-flag or warning sign for further inquiry about unresolved grief, moral injury, and/or unresolved trauma. Is the blame for something actually done (such as intentionally hurting someone), or for actions they wished they had done? There is a difference. Moral injury is the distress of doing actions that are against one's morals, such as killing in war. Moral injury requires its own version of healing self-blame, discussed in Chapter 9. This is a different type of blame than an abuse survivor blaming oneself for not escaping abuse. Abuse is an action perpetrated by someone else, who chose to do what was done. *Warrior Renew* (Katz, 2014) discusses putting blame where blame is due and letting others be responsible for their own actions. Abuse survivors may regret certain choices and behaviors. They may feel angry about what happened and may grieve losses. But it is impossible to be at fault for one's own abuse. Regardless of what they did or didn't do (e.g., scream, or fight harder), that does not cause someone to violate another person.

For example, let's say Adam is at his friend's house and he puts his wallet on the table, with a $100 bill in it. Is a theft happening? No. It requires a thief for a theft to occur. Someone would need to reach in and take the money, and then try to get away without getting caught. Even if one argues that the wallet shouldn't have been on the table, if a thief was looking to steal, they would find a way. If there was no thief, it wouldn't matter where the wallet was placed. It takes the actions of a thief for a theft to occur. Similarly, the one who abuses is the one who is at fault for the abuse. To grasp this concept, it requires stepping outside of one's experience. It requires considering the thief, their motive, and intention. This can be particularly challenging for children because they lack perspective, or any other way to make sense of something that does not make sense. However, when put into a story, or metaphor such as the wallet on the table, people can quickly realize that it is not the wallet's fault, and not theirs either. This insight changes the narrative and reshapes the neural network.

Virtual reality goggles

People are motivated to try to make sense of their experience and in so doing construct a framework to explain it. Based on their experiences, they learn that, "Oh, this is how the world is... and this is who I am..." Future experiences then weave together a narrative that becomes the implicit backdrop for anticipating, expecting, interpreting, and responding to the world.

A metaphor to explain the influence of the past on being present is to imagine everyone is wearing a pair of virtual reality goggles. The goggles filter how people anticipate, perceive, interpret, and respond to the present. What is playing on the inside of the goggles is the accumulation of past experiences, influencing interactions with present reality. These are sophisticated goggles and can change with one's mood. Similar to photochromic lenses that are transparent indoors and darken to sunglasses when exposed to ultraviolet light from the sun, these goggles are sensitive to emotions and may alter the filter of one's perceptions, especially if a familiar emotional neural network is activated.

If these goggles are always there, where the past is ready to filter the present, then how does one become free of the influence of the past? Can we take off the virtual reality goggles? Maybe not completely, but we can change the filter by resolving the past, practice being present, and upgrading the lenses.

Like wearing a pair of virtual reality goggles, experiential holograms are the implicit lens for expecting, interpreting, and reacting to the world.

Chapter summary

This chapter explains how memories of the past link together and influence the perception of the present. It discusses associative learning and more specifically how memories associate through emotions. The metaphor of a string of holiday lights is offered to explain how memories link to an emotion. Other metaphors are discussed such as addressing the relationship blueprint instead of particular relationships. Self-blame is also discussed as a common narrative for making sense of a trauma experience. The past becomes a filter, like wearing virtual reality goggles through which we anticipate, perceive, and respond to life events.

Chapter 4

Holograms and experiential holograms

This chapter discusses the model of a hologram for understanding emotional and interpersonal patterns. Holograms have unique aspects such as how the whole is encoded within the parts, and how holograms appear real but are projections from holographic film. The chapter will explain how holograms are made and why this is a plausible model for understanding repeating patterns in people's lives.

Case example: Who's first, the cat or me?

Ariana, a highly educated Caucasian lesbian woman in her late forties started off our session telling me that the only way she made it through the week was knowing she could come here today to express her pent-up frustration. The problem is when her partner comes home, instead of having intimate time with her, her partner says, "after I pet the cat." Apparently, when she is gone all day, she is concerned that her cat would feel abandoned. Ariana was so hurt and outraged. She said to me, "Why does she always have to pet that stupid cat first?" She quickly stated that she knows it is "all her own issue" and "if she could only be more accepting, everything would be better."

I wanted to know more about her experience. I asked her to tell me what she was feeling. She responded that she felt hurt and angry and that she should be able to handle this better. She continued to speak intellectually about her addictions to cigarettes and food. She said that smoking was a way to "numb the heart chakra." She quoted information she learned in Alcoholics Anonymous (AA) about acceptance. I knew I had to redirect her back to her feelings. I asked her how she felt when her partner pets the cat. She said, "I feel jealous and angry." "What else?" I asked. She said, "fear that I am being left out." I asked her where she felt her fear and then to put her hand over the spot. She had her hand on her stomach. I asked her to feel the sensations and describe the shape and color of her fear. She described it as a ball the size of a golf ball and it was red and orange and yellow. We did the same procedure with her anger and she put her hand on her intestine/

DOI: 10.4324/9781003223429-5

bowel area. She described it as hot smoldering coals. She stated that she did not want to spend too much time feeling anger because it was a "high" for her. She stated she was addicted to anger and could get stuck in it. She described how it was reinforced and justified by feelings of self-righteousness and indignation. I asked what would cool the area and she said she already threw a bucket of ice over it and it was giving off steam. She did the same for her fear and it loosened from a ball to flesh-colored silly putty.

Then we went to her heart. She had mentioned she dramatically increased her smoking over the past week and related this to "protecting her heart chakra." I was curious to find out what she was feeling in her heart. She placed her hand on her heart and described a beautiful iridescent pulsating heart. However, when we talked about it being warm and full, she said it varied and seemed to have cycles of being warm and cold. I asked, "how does your heart feel when your partner pets the cat? She replied, "It's afraid it is not going to get her attention." I probed, "like there wouldn't be enough left over for you?" She said, "Yes, and my little girl is having a temper tantrum!" She chastised herself and accused herself of being petty and not accepting enough. I recognized that this was the entry to her experiential hologram. I hypothesized that when she was a little girl, she had a temper tantrum about something and was expected to be quiet and accept her circumstances. I was curious about this hypothesis and if it related to her feelings with her partner. I asked about her little girl and if this situation seemed familiar to her. She revealed that she has a sister that is 11 months younger than her. Her mother would always rock her to sleep first. My client stated she felt left out and competitive with her sister for her mother's attention. She stated she felt neglected in general by her mother who was a practicing alcoholic. But even more painful was watching her attend to her younger sister (and not her). She stated she always felt like the number two child in the family even though she was older.

She explained how all her life she has used her addictions to fill her empty heart. Now, she is wanting her partner to do the same. We discussed that this is a reminder to work on soothing herself, reminding herself that she is loved, and connecting with her own "higher power" (a concept frequently used in AA). We also discussed how her partner is limited and unable to fulfill her. She said her higher power is limitless and can provide as much love as she is open to receiving. She put her hand back on her heart. I asked her to think of a symbol she can use when she sees her partner petting the cat to remind her about her own self-soothing or self-love. This coupled with slow deep breathing helped regulate her emotions. I asked her how she felt at the end of this session. She said it always takes her some time to process when she has had an important break-through.

During our fourth session, she announced that after therapy, she and her partner were going to pick up a kitten just for her. I thought this was a creative solution. Now they can tend to their cats, together. This client had certain therapeutic structures in place before she came to meet with me. She speaks AA language. I did not challenge this, but rather took the position of being a visitor in her experiential world. Within the context of her experiential system, we worked on making the modifications so that she can construct a more adaptive concept of her childhood experiences of neglect. She considered new ways of making sense of her experiences by considering context from the perspective of other people who were involved. Then we discussed if she could meet her younger self, what would she say or do? She enjoyed the imagery reprocessing where her current age self visited her younger self to offer perspective, soothing, and reassurance. She said she realized she has been ignoring her inner little girl and wants to continue to communicate with her. At the end of her therapy, Ariana reported a marked improvement in her relationship, her little girl was more at peace, and she stated she had a transformative experience.

Holograms

In this case example, Ariana had an emotional response to her partner diverting her attention from her to the cat. She was aware on an intellectual level that it didn't change her partner's level of love for her. Yet, experientially it triggered deep overwhelming distress. Using associative principles relating her current emotions to her past, she was able to recall her childhood experience. She felt the old feelings of being disregarded while her mother attended to her younger sister. She felt ignored and insignificant, and she personalized this to mean that she didn't matter. This belief has been playing in the background of her mind ever since. Like the virtual reality goggles metaphor, her perception of herself became the filter through which she anticipated, interpreted, and reacted to life events. She was reacting to her partner, but also reacting to many incidents of neglect, stemming from the formative experiences with her mother (and sister). Like the string of holiday lights metaphor, neglect was the string that got plugged in, and it lit up all related experiences.

What was activated was more than a cognition, belief, or perception, but rather a visceral emotional reaction. It was experiential, and felt very real. But like a hologram that appears real, is actually a projection from her past. Similar to the metaphor of addressing the blueprint (the source of the feeling), therapy focused on the source of the distress inside Ariana. Had the therapy focused on changing the partner's behavior, or addressing Ariana's symptoms, the issue could likely surface again with someone else, or in another situation.

The hologram is used as a model to explain the phenomena of a pattern of re-emerging experiences in people's lives. A hologram is a three-dimensional image produced by splitting a laser beam so that one half is projected onto an object and then onto photographic film, while the other half of the laser beam, called the reference beam, is bounced off of a mirror then to the object and then to the film. When the two laser beams meet on the photographic film, the light waves hit almost simultaneously, and form an interference pattern. This is like dropping a pebble in a pond and then dropping a second pebble in the same pond. The two pebbles create a series of concentric circles that overlap. The photographic film records this interference pattern and the image is embedded within the pattern. When the film is waved, there appears to be a three-dimensional image that is projected into space. If a piece of the film is broken off, the whole image can still be projected. The resolution may diminish, but each part of the film contains information about the whole. Also, there is an integrity within a system as each part carries consistent patterns or isomorphic themes throughout the layers within a system. An isomorphic theme is the pattern that is repeated throughout a system.

Holograms are made by a process where an image is recorded on to an interference pattern so that the whole image is embedded in every part of the film.

The hologram is used in this theory because of three unique qualities. First, a hologram creates a three-dimensional image that appears to project into space. It looks real but is actually a projection from the film. People can react to the hologram as if it is real but it is actually an illusion. It is a projection from a holographic film. Second, a piece of the holographic film contains the whole image. Thus, each part contains information about the whole and the whole contains information about the parts. Each piece (or in this case experience) is a whole unto itself, as well as a part of a greater whole in a given context. In other words, each relationship encodes information about a whole relationship pattern. When a client shares an upsetting interpersonal interaction, they are revealing elements about their whole life. The whole is embedded in the parts. Finally, holograms have integrity created by consistent themes that are repeated throughout the layers in a system. There is consistency, so much so, that people are not even aware they are replicating themes in their lives. They believe their holograms are real, and they believe their experience is their reality.

- Holograms are an illusion that appears to be real/projected from the film
- The whole is contained in the parts
- There are consistent themes that run throughout a system which maintains the integrity of the system. This is called isomorphic organization

Holographic memory

Does the brain really process information like a hologram? Since the hologram is used in this model, it seems appropriate to at least attempt to answer this question. What I can glean from the literature is that this is a very complex, controversial topic, and that research is still evolving. One of the early pioneers in this field was Karl Lashley (1929) who demonstrated in rats that learning is distributed across all parts of the brain rather than stored in a single region. He trained them to do certain tasks, and then after removing sections of their brains, he found they retained their training. Paul Peitsch (1981) conducted similar studies with salamander brains and concluded that Lashley's (and later Karl Pribram's) claim that memories do not have a specific location in the brain was correct. Another pioneer is John Eccles who was a neurophysiologist who described how a wave could be generated at the branching ends of presynaptic axons. These waves could create interference patterns in the brain. Pribram (2007) hypothesized that the brain may use holographic principles where memory may be stored on these interference patterns and then it can recreate that information when activated. Pribram suggests these processes involve electric oscillations in the brain's fine-fibered dendritic webs, which are different from the more commonly known action potentials involving axons and synapses.

Since experience occurs with multisensory inputs that trigger firing of various neurons simultaneously, this too could create interference patterns. This may be how we can store vast amounts of information that we encounter on a daily basis. Some research suggests that memories are encoded throughout the brain in this manner. Pribram (2007) outlines his current thinking regarding holonomic brain theory and some common misconceptions leading to inaccurate statements such as the brain itself is a hologram; rather, it can use holonomic principles for storing and retrieving memory.

Dennis Gabor won the 1971 Nobel Prize in Physics for his work on holography. He found that he could use Fourier transformations to convert images to waveforms and then back into images. Using this mathematical formula, it was proven that the visual cortex cells respond to the waveform images created by the Fourier translations of the original images instead of to the original images. In other words, vision was found to respond to waveforms, as was found similarly in the ear (by Hermann von Helmholtz) and for smell, touch, taste, and movement. Fourier translation formulas were used to predict how people would respond to various frequencies in all of the senses. Thus, the brain appears to use Fourier transformations to analyze tasks and absorb them as a whole. In Pribram's holonomic theory, a piece of a long-term memory is similarly distributed over a dendritic arbor so that each part of the dendritic network contains all the information stored over the entire network.

Based on these functions, memory is not piecemeal (i.e., remembering only the smell of pumpkin pie) but rather it is holistic (i.e., the smell of pie is associated with sensations, Thanksgiving, sights, feelings, gustatory memories, etc...). Given that experience is encoded simultaneously and holistically, then it makes sense that if one part of an experience is recalled, then other parts are also recalled.

However, the opposite may also be true. The single neuron theory (also known as the Jennifer Aniston neuron theory, Halle Berry neuron theory, or grandmother cell) demonstrated that we have a specific neuron that reacts to images of a particular actress. This is an extreme version of the idea of sparseness. The opposite of the single neuron theory is the distributed representation theory that states that a specific stimulus is coded by its unique pattern of activity over a large group of neurons widely distributed in the brain. So is memory a single neuron, part of a network, located in a specific region, or diffusely spread throughout the brain? Likely there are multiple processes occurring. Pribram (2007) discussed deep and surface structures of memory that may explain some of these contradictory findings.

Bryukhovetskiy (2015) similarly discussed different communication processes: vertical communication from the nervous system (major organs) to the brain via pulses sent through axons of neurons (neural tissue), and horizontal complex communication. He stated that "hologram formation is a key mechanism of horizontal complex commutation.... holograms are transported by the natural flow of CSF (cerebrospinal fluid), permitting long-distance transfer of information and communication between various brain regions" (Bryukhovetskiy, 2015). He asserts that the pia mater, the delicate innermost layer of the meninges which surrounds the brain and spinal cord, is where memory is stored holographically. The management, processing, and storage of information is performed in the CSF around the brain and the pia mater is a "unique anatomical substrate for the recording, storage, and reproduction of information." This supports the distributed memory theory and would explain Lashley's and Peitshch's findings (since the pia is outside of the grey matter of the brain). While Bryukhovetskiy (2015) clearly stated that long-term memory is the basic function of the pia, we cannot exclude the more traditional models of neural networks. More research is needed to understand the relationships between the pia and neural networks of the nervous tissue. Furthermore, there are different types of long-term memory including implicit and explicit memory, as well as memory distributed throughout the body such as muscle memory or physical memories that may occur after a trauma. Since CSF runs throughout the body, linking body to brain, perhaps this is a conduit consistent with Bryukhovetskiy's (2015) ideas.

The neuroscience of memory is exceedingly complex and beyond the scope of this book. Nonetheless, perhaps cognitive-experiential theory (CET) can help explain some of the contradictory processes. Epstein (2014) suggests that the cognitive-rational system relies heavily on verbal memory. Examples are solving mathematical problems, remembering items on a grocery list, and remembering numbers, words, and names. In contrast, the experiential system relies heavily on visual-sensory processes including experiential beliefs, implicit awareness, and impressions, as well as recalling memories of experiences, vicarious experience, and fantasy. The experiential system activates emotions and physical sensations. It would not be surprising if there were distinct neural processes for the two types of thinking delineated in CET.

Experiential exercise 1: Imagine recalling a place where you grew up as a child. Perhaps, close your eyes and remember your home, moving from room to room, recalling as many details as you can. Imagine being there—like an exact holographic replication.

Experiential exercise 2: Imagine sitting on a warm sandy tropical beach looking out at the ocean. It is a warm sunny day, the sky is blue; imagine feeling the warmth of the sun on your face, smelling and tasting the salty air, listening to the waves, running your fingers through the soft warm sand. You can imagine being there, as if in a holographic replication.

Experiential thinking, using imagery, can be helpful for problem solving and planning by imagining being in a situation and noticing what is needed. Furthermore, experiential-based thinking relying on one's own holographic recall may be particularly useful for social awareness, processing how others are feeling (by decoding tone of voice, facial expression, and body posture), as well as unspoken communication of intention, motives, or sarcasm, and hidden meanings. The mental construct of self in relationship with others is known as *mentalization*. Fonagy (2002) defined mentalization as the ability to be aware of one's internal mental states, and to reflect on the thoughts, feelings, and intentions of others. Later, the definition included the ability to represent mental states or hold a mental image of oneself and imagine how relationships may unfold (Allen & Fonagy, 2006). Mentalization describes the ability to put oneself in another's position (e.g., as if one were in their shoes). This ability utilizes experiential thought to imagine how others would feel, or how they might feel if they were in another's circumstance. For most, this ability is not effortful, but rather an automatic social skill, and could tap into one's social-emotional holograms which facilitates efficient processing to recall similar feelings in order to empathize and relate to other people's experience. Drawing upon one's own experience enables one to imagine how someone else would feel, or how they might feel in another situation. This supports emotional resonance, and empathy. Mentalization is not a language-based process but is rather experiential-based (visual-sensory). Automatic experiential thinking is deeply rooted in our biology, part of our social-functioning, and as Epstein (2014) states, guides our daily operations.

A limitation of mentalization is that it assumes others feel the same way as the perceiver. If you imagine being in a situation, the reference point is still you. Perhaps someone else would not feel the same way. Thus, even with this important skill, one can be stuck in one's own perceptions and may lack a perspective only seen outside of oneself. This is an added component of holographic reprocessing—as it supports considering context, perceptions from another's point of view (distinct from oneself), and from a broad meta-point of view (discussed in Chapter 10).

To summarize this discussion, memory and neural-cognitive processes are complex and may include holographic phenomena. While neuroscience of the brain is beyond the scope of this book, what is relevant is the *practical application of the hologram* to increase awareness, resolve old limiting patterns, and address automatic trauma holograms. Emotionally significant experiences can influence perceptions both at the surface and in deep implicit ways. The issue is always there, like waves rumbling beneath the surface. The hologram is a compelling model to communicate these ideas. It provides a holistic way of conceptualizing complex psychological processes. When brought fully into awareness, people may feel a sense of relief, validation, and resonance that it makes sense to them. In this therapy, the hologram is used as a model to explain an observed phenomenon that is not linear but rather holistic. It describes how one emotional experience can contain a whole pattern, just like a hologram. The consistency across experiences is isomorphic, just like a hologram. The belief in something that feels real, but is actually an illusion, like a projection from a film where the film is the past, is also just like a hologram. These observations fit remarkably well with the holographic model. And in time, we may come to better understand holonomic processes in our human physiology.

There are other concepts that are also compelling, like David Bohm's ideas of holomovement and implicit and explicit order, as well as non-local communication, entanglement, and quantum mechanics—all very interesting concepts and worth further inquiry, but are beyond the scope of this text. Nonetheless, they suggest that there are many layers of reality—some that we are aware of, and others that we are not. For this reason, further inquiry is intriguing and consistent with holographic reprocessing's goal to seek to understand our multi-layered perceptions of reality.

Client quote: "The experience of discovering my hologram helped me a lot. I was able to discern why I have issues with rejection—very enlightening."

Experiential holograms

Experiential hologram refers to a theme of experiences that re-emerge throughout a person's life. The consistent patterns are isomorphic themes that repeat through time and in various contexts. Experiential holograms are formed during emotionally-charged or traumatic events. Forming these holograms can have an important adaptive function to alert people to mobilize and protect themselves in dangerous or emotionally difficult situations. In the case example at the beginning of this chapter, Ariana's experiential hologram is an interpersonal one of feeling left out and ignored. It is a painful hologram that originated from her past experiences. The current event with her partner brought her background feelings to the foreground. The hologram is always there, consistent over time, and may activate across relationships and in various situations. Ariana had already spent time reflecting on her life, analyzing her feelings, and confronting negative thinking. It did not require too much for her to make the connections with her past. But she still feared being left out, and interpreted her partner's behavior to mean that she was not loved. Thus, it was a replaying of her past in the present. One of the benefits of this model is since the experiential hologram is always present, it can reveal itself in any significant relationship or experience—either in the present, past, or distant past. This gives therapists incredible flexibility. Whenever clients discuss something of emotional significance, the hologram is likely rumbling beneath the surface.

For Ariana, current events activated her beliefs that she is "always ignored, left out, and second." She personalized the experience and believed it means that she is unloved (by her mother, and now her partner). Her perceptions are the result of her attempt to make sense and cope with her experience. While something bad is happening, the person in the situation is actively coping and reacting. It's only after the fact, once out of the active danger, that they may reflect and wonder why this happened to them, and what does it mean about them? Furthermore, they wonder, what could they have done to have avoided the outcome or to avoid having the experience again? At some level, it seems prudent to reflect on past traumas to try to make sense of the experience. But if the reflection leads to a conclusion of global culpability (e.g., "It's my fault because of who I am"), then how can one control an outcome if the person is part of the issue? It is similar to a dog chasing its own tail.

For example, Jake feels rejected and concludes that he is not good enough. He makes concerted efforts to be perfect, and to be better than perfect by exceeding expectations. Theoretically, this should resolve the feeling of not being good enough and then, he'll be accepted. If he is outstanding, then he won't feel rejected. However, it is not only impossible because he will always find ways where he could do more or be better, but he becomes his own worst critic, judging whether or not he is good enough. He is in his own holographic trap, and none of it actually addresses the issue of his feeling rejected. Someone else rejected him because of their own issues, not because of Jake. Jake believes it is because he is not good enough and that remains his belief, regardless of what he is able to achieve. Running faster on the hamster wheel does not get a person any closer to their goal. In fact, the only way to free oneself from the hologram is to get off of the wheel. This will be discussed in detail in future chapters.

Experiential holograms are holistic imprints not only of images and sensations of significant past experiences, but they also include an experiential narrative about the meaning that one attributes to the experience. This is the personalization of what it means about oneself, others, and the world. It is an implicit cognitive-emotional heuristic. It is a concrete, categorical conclusion such as, I am not "good enough," "worthy enough," I'm "gullible," "bad," etc. This is the global attribution heuristic as mentioned earlier, where one attributes poor outcomes to oneself.

Situations, people, or events in the environment may trigger the activation of an experiential hologram. For example, a difficult relationship with someone's boss could be the perfect environmental context to project an experiential hologram of previous difficult relationships with an authoritarian spouse or partner, or abusive parent. The experiential hologram becomes a re-enactment of previous experiences. Because certain outcomes are expected, people interpret and respond according to their expectations. This prompts others in the situation to respond to these responses. Thus, the original expected outcomes are often realized. Experiential holograms are activated, re-enacted, and then reinforced through new experiences confirming the original hologram. Although someone may project a past experience on to a new situation, it is not exactly the same. Aspects may be the same, expectations and responses may be the same, but there is a living, interactive quality to the new experience. It is like walking on to the *Star Trek* television series (Abrams, 2009) holo-deck where the hologram and live human-being interact.

Experiential holograms have no sense of time. The experiential system does not process information in a linear manner, so time as a concept does not exist in the experiential mind. Thus, if a traumatic event occurred 30 years ago and an experiential hologram is activated, the sensations of trauma could be experienced in the present time, similar to as they were in the past. Without awareness, or conscious effort, people may rely on automatic processing and repeat the same set of responses. They may experience being stuck in a repeating holographic pattern, reinforcing limiting beliefs instead of resolving them.

Replaying holograms can be either re-traumatizing and reinforcing, or an opportunity to learn and change the pattern. Each new experience becomes an opportunity to rewrite or rescript the holographic pattern. In the case example at the beginning of this chapter, Ariana is aware of her hologram and can actively confront and disengage from old feelings. Each time, she disengages from feelings of being left out and reaffirms her connection, she changes the pattern. In this way, life becomes the stage for the re-enactment and also the resolution of experiential holograms. Because the experiential mind has no sense of time, a disconfirming experience in the present confuses old holographic patterns and begins to build new associations, and new learnings.

Formation of experiential holograms

As discussed, we are motivated for cognitive efficiency. As such, we rely on heuristics and automatic responses to quickly and efficiently direct our everyday functioning. As we develop (from infancy), we learn to recognize and anticipate interactions with others. We develop a perception of self, based on those interactions. This is consistent with the attachment literature. Attachment theory focuses on internalized perceptions of how people feel about themselves in relationships, such as feeling secure (trusting and safe) versus insecure (anxious, avoidant, or disorganized) as a basic foundation in relationships. Attachment is distilled to this: Do people have a secure or insecure working model of self and self in relationships with others? In attachment-based therapy, the goal is to internalize an improved feeling of security. Holographic reprocessing, delineates several components to the patterns. This includes triggering experiences, perceptions of self, coping strategies (avoidant and compensating), motivation to meet unmet needs, and residual emotions. In other words, it is a dynamic pattern that includes how people interpret and interact with others. These patterns develop based on how the person perceives how they were treated by others, and the conclusions they draw based on their perceptions. For example, if people experienced parental neglect, rejection/criticism, betrayal, or endangerment, what does this mean about them? Are they unimportant, not good enough, gullible, or unsafe? People interpret and make sense of their perceived experiences by thinking it is about them, their fault, and the basis of their worth. Once internalized, they may anticipate that others will continue to treat them in the same fashion into the future. In addition, they may have chronic feelings such as anxiety, anger, feeling wary or apprehensive, or sad/depressed, and may develop a variety of coping strategies including avoidance of painful or uncomfortable feelings, and compensating strategies to try to meet basic needs. Basic emotional and interpersonal needs may include feeling loved, attended to, having self-esteem, and security (Janoff-Bulman,1992; Epstein, 2014). Holographic reprocessing adds to previous models, including attachment theory, by delving into the source of the pattern, and particularly the personalized meaning attributed to the experience.

In this chapter's case example, Ariana perceived that she was unimportant because her mother chose to care for her sister first. Attachment focused therapies may work on helping Ariana internalize feeling loved and valued to improve her anxious insecure attachment to a more secure one. However, her perception about what happened may not be accurate in the first place! Perhaps her mother viewed Ariana as the strong one who didn't need the same attention as her more vulnerable younger sister. Maybe her mother relied on Ariana to be more mature because her mother knew her younger sister had emotional issues. Maybe her mother saw Ariana's strengths and had to deal with her own deficits. In a bigger picture, her mother's preoccupation with alcohol may have allowed Ariana to be more independent, and maybe her upset with her mother was the reason she sought therapy, specifically to find ways to not be like her mother. There are many possible interpretations and aspects of her experience to explore. Ariana's conclusion (that she is somehow not important because of her perception of how her mother treated her) is the culprit (the blueprint, the holographic film) perpetuating a falsehood about her. It's this personalization (e.g., perception that because mother chose her sister first, that it means she is not important) which creates the experiential hologram. If the perception never changes, then this belief is held intact. Holographic reprocessing adds the element of addressing meaning-making to people's experience. This is one of the main targets in this treatment. This coupled with self-soothing skills, and imagery reprocessing to meet her younger self's unmet needs, changes the experiential hologram.

> Experiential holograms develop as a means to efficiently process interpersonal relationships, traumas, and significant events. It is a cognitive heuristic that resides in the experiential system.
>
> The personalization of events (what this means about me) is a way to make sense of oneself and the world. People develop coping strategies consistent with their personalized beliefs to secure basic needs of life including love, attention, affection, self-esteem, and security. This is how the hologram forms—to efficiently process information, avoid pain, and secure basic needs.

Much of the discussion has been about experiential holograms formed in relationships; however, in response to traumatic or emotionally significant experiences, people may develop experiential holograms due to unresolved guilt and/or grief, personalizing self-blame, or other persistent negative or limiting self-perception ("it's my fault," "I'm no good," etc.). Examples include moral injury (guilt and blame for acting in ways that go against one's morals and ethics), complicated grief (blame and regret from unresolved grief or losses), and trauma-based holograms developed from events such as abuse, medical trauma, natural disasters, or accidents (with lingering self-blame, fear, anger, etc.). The replaying of the past is very much alive in a person's psyche, unlike other memories that seem to fade away as a distant memory from the past.

Experiential holograms

- They are a pattern of perceptions/experiences of self or self in relationship with others that is consistent over time and across relationships (understanding one relationship, means understanding the whole).

- They are an implicit theory of self and others (largely unconscious but rumbling in the background) and different circumstances bring it forward.
- Clients may not be aware or able to report them, but once made explicit, seem to resonate with experiential relief.
- They may also develop in response to traumatic or emotionally significant experiences, and include coping strategies to avoid pain—but usually sets the person up for recapitulation; hence, lead to a feeling of being stuck.
- They become deeply embedded in one's conceptual system. Self-evident and self-validating. For example, "I always feel this way so it must be true... this is my reality."

Trauma triggers versus experiential holograms

While both a trauma trigger and an experiential hologram may be activated by something in the current environment that reminds one of the past, they are distinct. A trauma trigger is recalling a specific experience activating the automatic response to protect from threat or danger. A trauma trigger sends off an alarm and the associated neuro-chemical mechanisms activate the fight, flight, or freeze response. A trauma trigger means "sound the alarm to protect against danger." Physiologically, the experience is sudden, intense, and physical. The reaction peaks and then subsides. Some experience it as anxiety, or a panic attack. Others may worry that they are having a heart attack. A trauma trigger may be a reaction to something specific or may become triggered without the person consciously knowing why. A trauma trigger may also be a sudden recollection of a past trauma experience including feelings of grief, disgust, horror—it is a replaying of a trauma memory. The trauma memory may grab one's attention, bring up old feelings, and then fade away.

An experiential hologram, on the other hand, involves a complex and persistent system including ongoing perceptions about the self and others, as well as coping strategies, avoidance strategies, and motivations to meet unmet needs. The experiential hologram is deeper and more integrated into the personality. It may be a guiding factor played out in a variety of relationships, especially romantic relationships. It may activate a variety of emotions such as anger, fear, jealousy, hurt, or loneliness as well as cognitions (e.g., assumptions, meanings, interpretations), and coping reactions. It is an automatic reaction that reinforces one's perception of their reality including perceptions about oneself, others, and interactions.

A trauma trigger is a sudden reminder of danger, horror, or disgust, activating the autonomic nervous system alarm system to mobilize for protection. The person may feel a sense of disorientation as a result of a sudden flood of stress hormones. Activating the emergency system is a biological response that both humans and animals have as a protective measure to ensure survival. The stress and associated emotions peak and subside.

An experiential hologram activates holographic images/sensations that are projected on current relationships and experiences, includes perceptions, attributions and meaning about oneself and others. It is the on-going assumptions playing in the background of one's mind. It is complex and persistent. It is a filter through which people anticipate, perceive, interpret, and respond to life experiences.

Chapter summary

Experiential holograms are: 1) experiential because they are formed by experience and reside in the experiential system (e.g., implicit, and emotional); 2) holographic because it feels real, but the personalized perception is actually an illusion of truth, a belief, but not necessarily the truth. Just because someone experienced betrayal, neglect, being taken advantage of, criticized, abused, etc., in the past, does not mean that it was because of them, or who they are, or that it has to continue to be that way. People tend to make sense of their experience by personalizing it to mean something about them.

Part 2

Implementing holographic reprocessing

Chapter 5

Initial session and preparation for therapy

This chapter discusses the initial session for case conceptualization, presenting rationale, and overview of the therapeutic steps for holographic reprocessing. Each therapeutic step includes a description of the associated metaphors and strategies used for implementation.

Case example: It was not her fault

Abigail was a self-assured 33-year-old Hispanic woman. She was referred to the clinic because she told her primary care provider that she was angry and wondered if this was depression. She was very reluctant to get involved with therapy. She said she was a successful manager at her work and she earned a master's degree in engineering, and stated it is a very competitive field. During our first session, she was cold, judgmental, and critical of me. However, I quickly realized that her defensiveness was a symptom of how she was feeling inside. She was rejecting therapy, rejecting me, and yet stayed for the entire session to tell me how much she didn't need this. I understood she must be experiencing tremendous fear and was defending against being vulnerable. Instead of reacting to her, I breathed, non-defensively, inviting her to tell me what it's like for her at work (as this appeared to be a safe place for her). I could tell she had a lot of responsibility. I gave an empathic reflective statement that it was difficult working with others to get them to achieve like she would want them to. She agreed and seemed a bit more relaxed. I think she appreciated being heard. Then I put out an interpretation that it might be lonely being the manager and wondered if she had support? She paused, not sure if she wanted to reject the idea, or agree. Then she sighed as if to release her heavy armor. She acknowledged her frustration and loneliness. I could see emotion coming to the surface. We discussed anger and how it could potentially be related to depression as this was the referring question. She said the discussion made sense to her. She visibly looked more at ease. I introduced the concept of cognitive experiential systems and the idea of addressing the blueprint, not the houses, to heal issues that may

DOI: 10.4324/9781003223429-7

be playing out in various relationships. By the end of the first session, we had established a good working rapport; we completed the initial intake; and we agreed holographic reprocessing would be a good approach for her. She was motivated to engage.

We worked on emotion regulation, and I continued to listen to information that might reveal her experiential hologram. On the intake she denied trauma and didn't want to talk about her childhood. In the third session, she said she was ready to share a secret with me. She told me that her father molested her. She felt a lot of shame sharing this and the most painful part of the experience was her guilt. She said she encouraged him. Now she sees this as "sick" and can't tolerate how she contributed to this horrible event. She was angry at him, but confessed she was really angry at herself.

We discussed what happened and it became evident that she did indeed snuggle up with him. She liked his attention and it made her feel beautiful and special. However, she didn't realize the difference between attention, affection, and sex. She did not foresee what would happen to her. She felt violated, guilty, and ashamed. We used the age-comparison technique to help her see context. Her father was a bit older than she was now. She anchored herself to the here and now, practicing her slow deep breathing. She was able to shift the focus from what she did, to what the 36-year-old did. She was able to put blame where blame was due. He was the one who knew better. We acknowledged that he knew what he did was wrong. Of course he did, he was a 36-year-old man. She saw how he used her desire for attention to manipulate her and make her feel responsible for the act. She saw that she wasn't the guilty party. She saw that she was a normal girl who wanted to be loved. Her behavior may (or may not) have been inappropriate, but that was not the cause of the violation. Her behavior did not cause him to do what he knew was wrong. She also embraced a meta-reframe, from blaming herself for her mother's subsequent divorce from him (thinking she ruined their marriage), to seeing their divorce as a "blessing" and glad her mother got away from that "jerk" later to find a better partner.

In the reprocessing, she cried, and held the young girl in her arms and declared that she never needs to pursue affection like that anymore. In a three-month follow-up session, she stated she feels softer and gentler. She sees the power of being calm, staying open, and less defensive. It is easier to relate with others. She was appreciative of the therapy and said she couldn't have imagined how much happier she is now.

The initial session

As in all psychotherapy, participants are welcomed, invited to engage in therapy, are informed about limits of confidentiality, office policies, expectations for treatment, documentation of sessions, and general orientation as part of the informed consent process. Participants typically have a presenting issue of concern and this is acknowledged and stated as part of their goals for treatment.

Therapeutic stance

As a therapist, the stance in conducting this treatment is being authentic, concerned, and relatable. Appropriate humor can help people feel relaxed, and can build rapport. Demonstrating openness, Rogerian-style unconditional positive regard, and accurate understanding will also deepen rapport. Listening skills and conceptualization on the part of the therapist is a critical factor in this modality. This makes holographic reprocessing more challenging than routinely applying a protocol or tool, but also makes it a gratifying way to practice therapy. Each person is a mystery, a puzzle, a knot to figure out and unravel. Therapists use their intellect, mentalization skills, and clinical intuition to listen and conceptualize what is really going on.

The therapist's stance is important in this model as effective therapy relies on the willingness of clients to disclose and invite the therapist into their most private, sensitive, and painful aspects of themselves. It also requires openness on the part of the therapist to see, feel, and acknowledge the client. As in the case example with Abigail, she came in defensive and rejecting. It would be easy to react in kind, and that would sufficiently sabotage the therapy. Instead, the therapist remained calm, practicing her own affect management skills, and listened. The stance is compassionate but objective. While the client sent potential hooks to engage anger or defensiveness, the therapist did not attach to the hooks and did not engage with a defensive response. This initial exchange is a critical first step in building rapport, safety, and a therapeutic alliance.

The technique used in this example was to respond to underlying emotions. What she presented on the surface was dismissive and rejecting, but what she presented underneath the surface was fear. The therapist can use mentalization skills to feel what the client is really saying and call that forth. It is reading the emotional subtext, which typically is the real communication. Once this is articulated, clients usually feel a deep sense of relief and trust. With Abigail, the in-road was acknowledging her loneliness. This was an emotion she could acknowledge and tolerate. In fact, it turns out that it was the root emotion, driving the sexual trauma. She had a neglect interpersonal hologram as her foundation which made her vulnerable to an experience of sexual trauma, and subsequently she had a moral injury which was expressed through anger and rejection. She could not accept what she did and blamed herself. She was suffering from self-rejection, and achievements at work were not healing her pain. The underlying neglect hologram tied all the pieces together in a way that helped her see that she made *perfect sense.*

Another example of building rapport was seen in the case example of Faith in Chapter 2. The therapist's questions about how the client felt helped deepen the conversation to issues of abandonment. Notice, the conversation was not about the friend or about trying to argue her out of her feelings or perceptions about her friend (e.g., confronting all-or-nothing thoughts). This would keep the conversation superficial, likely frustrate the client, and lead to not feeling understood. Instead, the focus was on her emotions. Emotions are an efficient gateway to the implicit experiential system. Emotions about her friend led to emotions about her mother. The underlying issue was the same. The client was working on gaining awareness about her feelings of abandonment, her desire for reassurance, and ultimately a confirmation that she exists. The example ends with an exchange about whether or not Faith felt the therapist held her from week to week. She looked doubtful, but when it was turned back on her she said, "you got me." This could mean, "you caught me," or it could mean, "you understand me." In subtle ways throughout the interchange, the therapist was conveying the message, "I see you," "you exist."

Some conceptualization strategies

Patients typically identify their presenting problem as unwanted symptoms. Patients and providers are conditioned to label symptoms and view these as the target for intervention. Treatment plans often include goal setting to engage in activities to reduce symptoms. However, in holographic reprocessing, symptoms are not necessarily the target for treatment, but rather they are viewed as clues. They are the manifestation or response to an underlying unresolved issue. Symptoms develop in response to something. For example, anxiety is the body's response to perceptions of threat and danger. Worries are anticipating potential threat and danger. The body is responding to negative what-if scenarios and accordingly, feels anxious. Anxiety may be uncomfortable and something people want to reduce, but the focus of treatment, in this model, is the cause of the anxiety, not the anxiety itself. For example, if a patient presented with pain in their chest and their left arm, and these symptoms were addressed at face value, the patient might be sent to physical rehabilitation instead of monitored for a heart attack.

The therapist may ponder, why is this person having these symptoms? How could this response be adaptive? What is the underlying cause? The therapist would continue to wonder why these symptoms exist, until it makes sense. This is in contrast to cognitive approaches that confront and question the accuracy of a person's thinking and; therefore, the irrational nature of one's symptoms. In holographic reprocessing, symptoms are a rational response to an underlying perception that can best be understood through the experiential or emotional lens. By following an emotion, it can help reveal what is influencing the formation of the symptom. This facilitates deeper inquiry, understanding, and effective problem solving.

- How could a client's reactions be adaptive rather than pathological?
- How and why do the symptoms make sense?
- What is causing and maintaining the symptoms?

Example of symptoms as clues

Sally comes to therapy with a presenting problem of anxiety and emotional over-eating. She recently lost her job and she is appropriately worried about her rent. Sally says she can't keep a job because she is too anxious to work and asks for a letter to go on disability for her anxiety. She says she is unable to speak up for herself and calls herself "stupid." It is verified that Sally does have difficulty keeping jobs. She lost 5 jobs in the past 2.5 years. She tends to do well for a while, but becomes overwhelmed, her face turns red and she panics. She becomes so embarrassed that she doesn't return. She thinks she is in the wrong field. Other than work, she basically stays to herself, has a pet, a best friend, and is close to her family.

It would be reasonable to treat her anxiety including teaching coping skills, offering a referral for an evaluation for anti-anxiety medication, and to vocational rehabilitation to explore her career choices and possibly job retraining. It wouldn't be wrong to treat anxiety in this way. However, it may also be appropriate to find out more about Sally's story. In holographic reprocessing, we consider, why is she anxious, and in particular, why at work? What is she responding to and how is her response somehow adaptive?

Asking about her work, the emotions she feels, and situations that trigger anxiety, she realized she gets anxious around male authority figures. We linked her current experience to what might have happened in the past. She realized that work reminded her of the sexual assault she experienced by her superior in the military. At work, she feels threatened, hypervigilant, and worried of impending danger. She had never disclosed this to anyone before, nor has she dealt with her feelings. Anxiety prompted the behavior of running. She was running to be safe. She runs from jobs, but she is really running from fears of replicating past trauma.

Her symptoms were not the whole problem, but rather a *clue* of an underlying issue. She realized that she was avoiding work, running from uncomfortable situations, but she was not aware of why she was running. She did not link her current issues to the past. She was reacting to perceptions, likely implicit perceptions, that were activating reactions to threat and danger.

If the therapist could perceive life through their clients' virtual reality lenses, then they would know what the client was responding to. When therapists are presented with a client whose thinking, behavior, and decision making do not make any sense, then it is a clue that there is likely an experiential hologram in play. The person is responding to something from their past. On the surface, it may not make sense because others cannot see what they are responding to. An assumption in this treatment is that people do make sense, and it is the therapist's job to find out how.

Treatment assumptions

Holographic reprocessing assumes that people operate from a coherent conceptualization system that is motivated to conserve energy and function efficiently. As Kahneman and Traversky have articulated (Kahneman et al., 1982) we engage numerous cognitive heuristics or cognitive short-cuts to support efficient information processing. The experiential system consists of a vast network of associations to process, learn, and respond to life experiences in an efficient manner. To conserve energy, this network operates largely outside of our conscious awareness, automatically, without engaging the resource-draining rational-cognitive system.

Based on and as a result of this system, people experience consistent interpersonal patterns. Outcomes are self-evident, self-fulfilling, and self-regenerating. Thus, people tend to continue in a certain direction, creating similar relationships and interpersonal interactions. People are motivated by basic emotional needs such as wanting to feel loved, safe, and secure, and having the freedom to create and express themselves. This stems from a need for self-worth, as well as a desired belief in a world that is benevolent and meaningful (Janoff-Bulman,1992). These emotional needs also largely reside outside of conscious awareness to the extent that people may not be aware of what is driving their desires, impulses, and choices.

Holographic reprocessing assumes that everyone is already worthy of love, are good enough, deserving enough, important enough, etc., and these things are accessed internally not found externally. The belief of feeling otherwise is the holographic illusion. (Note: While there are possible exceptions, this statement is meant as a general statement for the majority of humanity.)

Holographic reprocessing is designed to be implemented flexibly and tailored to individual needs. It is meant as a way of conceptualizing issues. Once the conceptualization is clear, what is needed for treatment reveals itself. Some therapists, especially when starting their profession, may want to know what to do, and exactly what steps to follow, as if reading a recipe book. While this may be appealing for many reasons such as giving therapists a sense that they are doing it right, knowing what to do, sense of control, feeling effective, etc., following prescriptive protocols can inhibit deep listening, thwart creativity, and effectively miss the root issue. Instead, built into this therapy, is conceptualization. It includes inquiring about related issues, exploring formative causes, assessing for patterns, and then exploring curative factors such as considering context and meta-reframes. Nonetheless, a framework of steps is helpful as a guideline with the caveat that implementation should be tailored to the needs of the client.

Summary of the treatment process

This section provides an overview of the basic steps of holographic reprocessing with associated exercises for each step. Details of each will be presented in subsequent chapters.

Step 1. Gather information/build rapport/educate

The initial step includes establishing initial rapport, conducting a functional intake assessment to rule out risk factors, and establishing if this is an appropriate treatment for the client. It includes initial conceptualization efforts such as listening for patterns, and hypothesizing about types of experiential holograms. This is also the time to educate clients about the treatment: explain cognitive-experiential theory, how memories are organized by emotions (string of holiday lights metaphor), and that the treatment addresses underlying patterns, not specific events. This helps inform clients, deepens trust and understanding, and may motivate clients to engage. Most find it intriguing to learn about themselves, their patterns, and what is underlying their thoughts and behaviors. Most importantly, this step builds a therapeutic alliance where the client feels safe and is ready/able to invite the therapist into their experiential world.

Strategies used in this step:

- Listen, label, and bring forth people's emotions to facilitate understanding and rapport
- Explain cognitive-experiential theory
- Metaphor: What happens if when driving a car, the focus is on the rear-view mirror instead of the windshield?
- Metaphor: String of holiday lights to explain emotions and memory
- Metaphor: Treatment addresses blueprints, not particular houses, to get to the underlying unresolved issue

Step 2. Teach emotion regulation skills

The second step is learning emotion regulation skills. The extenT of the training is determined by client need. From the first session, clients may be taught these skills. Even if the session is almost over, take three to five minutes to teach the simple cleansing breath. This is helpful to initiate emotion regulation skills from the start. It gives clients a tangible tool that they can practice between sessions. The therapist can follow-up to find out if they used the tool, how was their experience? Or if they forgot, do they want a refresher? The therapist can write the tool on an index card and give it to the client. This reinforces learning, encourages commitment, and may give clients a sense that they are getting something useful from the treatment.

Depending on the level of dysregulation or need of the client, more or fewer skills are offered. This can help slow the process for those who may need more time to develop trust. Several strategies are offered in Chapter 6. As in all skills, first present the rationale of why it works, demonstrate how it works, and then invite the client to do it with the therapist.

Strategies used in this step:

- Rationale for emotion regulation (explain heart rate variability, what happens when the nervous system is dysregulated, how to reset one's baseline)
- Metaphor: for behavior change and addressing things that are working against oneself, like driving your car with the emergency-brake on
- Breathing: signal breath, cleansing breath, relaxation sandwich, slow deep breathing
- Grounding exercises: calming hand poses, grounding through feet, breath, diet choices
- Metaphors: Emotions flow through us like water flows through a hose, feelings peak and subside, like a wave they come and they go
- Metaphor: Washing machine to observe experience without getting caught up in it
- COPE strategy (cleansing breath, observation, positive self-talk, explanation)
- Healthy distraction strategies
- Positive focal point: a positive snapshot to rest one's mind (an image, song, prayer, smell, etc., that reminds the person of a positive or hopeful feeling)

Step 3. Identify patterns/formative causes of symptoms

In this step, more details are identified regarding the experiential hologram. This may include more in-depth conversation, or experiential discovery following emotions or body sensations to explore associations that may surface. Using the associative principle of the experiential system, present emotions can help the recall of similar past emotions to reveal patterns. This is a way to identify implicit beliefs about self and relationships. Gendlin's focusing procedure may be helpful for listening to one's inner-self. For interpersonal experiential holograms, various components may become apparent. Using the template of a pot on the stove may assist engaging a client in a conversation about components. The client and therapist work together to identify six components of the experiential hologram. This process is typically illuminating for clients. They are able to understand how their thoughts, feelings, and behaviors are part of a pattern, rather than random, or independent reactions. Clients typically have an "ah-ha" moment of awareness and appreciate the map of their pattern. *Note:* Not everyone will have or need a pot on the stove. This was originally designed for interpersonal experiential holograms. It is meant as a tool to help clients see themselves and their patterns. As with any tool, use as appropriate for each client.

Strategies used in this step:

- Metaphor: Virtual reality goggles to explain experiential holograms
- Discovery process: Attend to bodily cues/ encouraged emotional expression, use associations of present to past to reveal patterns, identify implicit beliefs about self and relationships; Gendlin's focusing exercise
- Journal exercise about relationship patterns
- Interpersonal Experiential Hologram Inventory
- Pot on the stove template
- Continued practice of emotion regulation skills
- Listening for core violations, personalized beliefs, residual emotions

Step 4. Consider context and other cognitive shifts

If not done already, this is the time to discuss vantage point and recalling memories. The metaphor of the observer vantage point (as the eagle) vs the field vantage point (as the field mouse) may be particularly helpful to set the stage for considering context. The observer vantage point facilitates considering context. This step is about reflection and viewing the event from various perspectives. The tissue box metaphor helps people consider multiple points of view such as seeing the situation from different sides of the box. This can include considering other people's agendas or motives; the perspective of time or age-comparison; or seeking a new understanding such as a meta-reframe that explains the event in an entirely new way. Context helps shift the event from the personal to the impersonal, promotes insight, and a broader contextually-based understanding. "Is there another way to understand this?"

Strategies used in this step:

- Metaphor: Eagle vs mouse to explain observer and field vantage points
- Metaphors and strategies to seeing multiple points of view:

- Metaphor: Tissue box to see multiple perspectives (consider other people's agenda and points of view)
- Age comparison to consider the ages of self and others at the time compared to one's current age
- Shrinking machine to reduce something big and scary to small and comical
- The book of norm, to see context, that others are responding to their own book of reality
- Hindsight advantage: knowing the outcome (e.g., you are going to survive)

- Meta-reframe to consider how an experience might make sense from a broad and inclusive way
- Several strategies to assist putting blame where blame is due to release responsibility for other people's choices and actions:

  - It takes a thief for a theft to occur
  - Catcher's mitt to toss back that which belongs to a perpetrator or someone else

- Strategy to disengage with anger and resentment due to injustice: Poetic justice that somehow, someway people reap their natural consequences
- Metaphor: The blue pen—you cannot change the color of the pen, just as we cannot change the past; this is to assist with acceptance of what is

Step 5. Imagery exercises

Imagery reaches the experiential system. Guided imagery to a nature scene (e.g., the beach) helps clients become more comfortable with imagery exercises. For releasing attachment to abuse, the catcher's mitt and shrinking machine are exercises to help disengage from fear and oppression. Imagery reprocessing is delivering a healing message to one's younger or traumatized self.

Preparation for imagery reprocessing may include writing a letter to one's younger self. This is to help the client process their feelings and integrate their understanding gleaned from considering context. Clients are trained how to recall a memory from the observer vantage point. When they are ready, they are assisted on a guided imagery exercise where they are to remain their current age and imagine meeting their younger self. They are asked, "What would you say? What would you do?" For interpersonal experiential holograms, one's current age self may address the underlying unmet need driving their hologram. For trauma, it may include communicating that what happened was not their fault. With grief, it may include imagining a conversation with the deceased, or engaging in imagery for release. It may include offering comfort, understanding, love, and/or attention (e.g., "You'll never be left alone again," "I'll protect you from now on,"

"Your needs matter"). After imagery reprocessing: clients are encouraged to take good care of their younger self, journal, breathe, rest, and drink water as they are doing deep emotional healing work. Some clients may wish to engage in multiple sessions of imagery reprocessing.

Strategies used in this step:

- Imagery: Catcher's mitt (toss negativity back to a perpetrator or place the negativity in a garbage can—"This is not mine")
- Imagery: Shrinking machine (imagine shrinking a threat to a small squeaky image)
- Imagery rescripting/reprocessing: When meeting one's younger self (future self, or deceased), what would you like to say, what would you like to do?

Step 6.Integration

The last step is integration, discussing closure, and how to move forward from this point. For some, once addressing the past, they are faced with another set of challenges on how to build their future. For others, once the past is complete, they are ready to end treatment. Clients are encouraged to reflect on their therapy experience and shift to a future-focused conversation. Clients may choose to write a letter to their future self, or engage in imagery to send a message to one's future self. A future focus may include discussing values, goals, being a contribution to others, and defining next steps in their life. They may accept a reframe to see potential triggers as an opportunity to flex their new skills and confront old patterns. Maybe at a time when they are vulnerable, they may interpret an interaction through old virtual reality goggles. Discussion about labeling it as their hologram, initiating slow deep breathing, and then considering context or evaluation from the eagle perspective can help. An imagery reprocessing booster session may also reinforce perspective and positive healing. Finally, clients are encouraged to welcome new activities with a positive attitude.

Strategies used in this step:

- Letter to one's future self
- Discuss values, goals, being a contribution
- Discuss addressing temporary relapses
- Reprocessing booster imagery if needed

Chapter summary

This chapter reviews the initial session of treatment, including the therapeutic stance, and goals for listening for patterns and underlying issues. The therapist can use mentalization skills to listen and feel what the client is saying beneath the surface to identify root emotions driving the pattern. Emotions are used as an efficient gateway to the implicit experiential system of processing to answer the question: "Why is this person having these symptoms?"

Six steps of holographic reprocessing

1   Gather information, build rapport, educate about the treatment
2   Teach emotion regulation skills
3   Identify patterns and formative causes of symptoms
4   Consider context
5   Releasing imagery or imagery reprocessing
6   Integration

Chapter 6

Emotion regulation skills

This chapter provides information for understanding and managing various emotions. It includes education and rationale for emotion regulation and provides exercises and metaphors. This is to bolster client's ability to detect and manage emotions.

Case example: Still fighting

Antonio came to therapy because he was feeling "down and anxious." He said he has lost his motivation. He had disrupted sleep and frequently dreamt of fist fighting. His wife urged him to get help because he had such fitful sleep that she made him sleep in the guest room. When asked about his fighting, he believed it had to do with his experiences in the military.

Antonio said his last year in the military was awful. He had a prior injury and his command was not supporting him with accommodations or leave for physical therapy. He said he knew they were targeting him and trying to get him out of the military. They kept setting him up for failure by raising the bar on qualifying tests. He said he was constantly feeling bullied and harassed by his First Sergeant. Nobody stood up to help him. He was trying to meet his own career goals and was frustrated because in spite of performing well, he was still harassed and discharged. He was also denied his last promotion and this really angered him.

He said he felt the harassment was because of racism and it isolated him from the team. He said he knows it was not his fault but still feels angry and hurt about it. What upset him most, was feeling pushed out of the military, against his will. Up until then, he had a perfect record, and did an exemplary job.

We gathered information and started to hone in on what upset him most. He was able to verbalize his frustration and pent-up anger. He felt this was a betrayal and was unjust. We discussed how treatment will help him disengage from his past so he can be present and move forward in his life. We also discussed taking slow deep cleansing breaths focusing on the exhale,

DOI: 10.4324/9781003223429-8

and creating a positive focal point. He said his life is so much better now, he has a better job, a happy marriage, and a good life. It didn't make sense to him why he was still so bothered about his past. He was hopeful and felt therapy would help him.

In the next session, Antonio said he was having dreams of fighting but not sure who he was fighting, then he woke up in a bad mood. He described that the bad dreams made him irritable for the rest of the day. He said it was unfair that they treated him this way with no consequences. We discussed the concept of *poetic justice* (that somehow, some way people reap the natural consequences of their own behavior). This is the concept that justice will be served in ways that we may not see. This offered him some relief.

We discussed that whatever happens to the First Sergeant, or any of the others, is their issue not his. His task is to release them from his path. His experience was validated and then we discussed the benefit to him to disengage from the past. He was encouraged to use his power to say, "no more," and not entertain thoughts of the past in his current life.

He also worked on slow deep breathing, using his positive focal point, and staying grounded and present. He wrote positive self-talk on a sticky note to post in his house to remind him to breathe.

By the third session, Antonio was able to articulate that what upset him most was feeling that he was a failure because he wasn't able to achieve what he wanted to. We discussed how this is his personalization of the experience. That *he* was a failure. This disregards all of his other achievements, and in reality, he didn't fail, his leadership failed him. He did a good job when he was there, and that is something to be proud of, and now that he is out, he can engage in the next phase of his life.

We discussed if he could meet his younger self what would he tell him? Now that he is out of the situation, he could look back on the past and see it from a new perspective. What does he want his younger self to know? He imagined his current age self telling his younger self, "You did a great job." He told his younger self that he was proud of him. He also told him that it's going to be much better when he leaves the military. He said, "You served your country even if you didn't leave on your own terms." And "Now your life is better." We reiterated that nothing can diminish the fact that he volunteered to serve his country, and he did a great job.

He said he would work on reminding himself of these things. I asked if there was anything else he needed to end the fight. He said in his dreams he wanted to speak but he couldn't. He said he got so upset that he just started fighting. But he said it is ineffective. Even talking about what happened got him choked up and frustrated. We discussed using the cleansing breath, taking a deep breath in through the nose and completely exhaling with a sigh. Then delivering his message, calmly. He practiced this while awake, and before he went to sleep, and it seemed to be working. He reported feeling more empowered and able to calm down.

Instead of fighting, his choice to disengage was a way to hold on to his power. He said that the discussion made sense to him. We discussed this is a different way to approach an abusive or inescapable situation. When he went on walks with his dog, he talked to his younger self (offering reassurance). He said it helps to remind himself that the military was over.

Not only was he taking ownership of his life, but he also made a powerful choice to disengage from thoughts of the past.

Emotion regulation

Holographic reprocessing includes several strategies for emotion regulation (e.g., affect regulation) to help people to mitigate, disengage from, or manage upset. Using skills can decrease the intensity, shorten duration, and perhaps lessen the frequency of bouts of emotional distress and trauma triggers. Affect management in and of itself, may not resolve past traumas, but may be an important, and for some, a necessary factor to promote change and healing. Several of the techniques presented in this chapter combine slow deep breathing with body awareness (interoceptive awareness). This may include a body scan or becoming aware of the sensations of the body.

It is well-established that chronic negative emotions and chronic stress can have a deleterious effect on health and well-being. Chronic negative emotions are related to a cascade of hormones such as elevated adrenaline and cortisol levels. Adrenaline increases heart rate and blood pressure. Cortisol increases sugars (glucose) in the bloodstream. To enhance resources in times of threat or danger, energy is redirected from nonessential functions such as the immune system, digestive system, reproductive system, and growth processes. This combined with potentially poor health behaviors could be a link associating chronic negative emotions and stress to more rapid aging, cardiovascular disease, osteoporosis, type 2 diabetes, arthritis, and some cancers due to the production of inflammatory chemicals in the body (Dhabhar, 2014; Power et al., 2020).

In addition, when trauma memories are triggered, and trauma images and sensations are suddenly recalled, it hijacks rational cognitive thinking (cortical inhibition), sending one's system into high alert. The perception of threat or danger takes precedent and activates the autonomic nervous system's alarm system to mobilize for protection. This activates the amygdala, the region in the brain that regulates the fight/flight/freeze response and the hypothalamic-pituitary-adrenal (HPA) axis. Multiple physiological reactions are activated—sending resources to the major muscles and essential functions to respond to threat and danger while reducing resources to nonessential functions such as higher cortical thinking. This is why when people are upset, they lose their ability to mentalize (consider how others may be feeling). This is usually in the context of perception of threat or danger, or high states of emotion such as anger, anxiety, or depression. This leads to a state of emotional dysregulation where people cannot access their higher cortical functioning. It disrupts logical thought or consideration of consequences. They lose a sense of empathy. They have a hard time making sense of other people's feelings and behavior, let alone their own. They become reactive, impulsive, and self-centered. This fuels categorical thinking (all or nothing), or narrow thinking leading to brooding and self-loathing.

The person is not necessarily in danger, but rather is responding to their perception of danger—and as such relies on implicit, automatic responses (without rational thought). Activating the emergency system is a biological response that both humans and animals have as a protective measure to ensure survival. But after trauma, the system may become too efficient, activating when it is not necessary. This is not only counter-productive and overwhelming, but potentially harmful to relationships, daily functioning, sleep, and well-being, leading to a cascade of other negative health consequences.

Those who recover more slowly from fight/flight/freeze responses may be more at risk for a variety of health conditions compared to those who recover more quickly (Ricard et al., 2014). A healthy amygdala dampens stress-induced activity of the HPA axis, which could have a protective influence on the cardiovascular, nervous, endocrine, and immune systems and play a role in maintaining physical health. Song et al. (2015) research found that individuals who had larger gray-matter volume in the amygdala reported not only a higher ability of emotion regulation but also better physical health. Gray-matter volume in the amygdala mediated the correlation between emotion regulation ability and physical health.

This chapter will present a variety of skills and practices to improve emotion regulation, and increase heart rate variability to improve responses to stress. State-level changes that are practiced and maintained for long periods of time have the potential to coalesce into more enduring trait-level changes (Hudson & Fraley, 2018). In other words, with practice, people can reset the baseline of their nervous system.

Regulating the autonomic nervous system

The body's autonomic nervous system is a dual system consisting of the sympathetic excitatory system and the parasympathetic inhibitory system. To assist remembering: Think of the sympathetic system as running up a hill and the parasympathetic system as parachuting to come down. The two systems work in tandem—communicating, regulating, and informing the nervous system. The inhale increases the heart rate and the exhale decreases the heart rate. The rate goes up and down with each full breath. Heart rate variability (HRV) is the fluctuation of time between heart beats. With an inhale the rate speeds up (less time between beats) and with the exhale it slows down (more times between beats). The time between heart beats can be mapped as up-and-down waves, ideally in a smooth consistent pattern with a long distance between the crest of the wave and the trough at the bottom of the wave.

Kim et al. (2018) reviewed studies that used HRV as a biomarker of stress and concluded that current neurobiological evidence suggests that HRV is a reliable factor impacted by stress. Those with chronic stress have hyperactivated sympathetic systems causing physical, psychological, and behavioral abnormalities, and low parasympathetic activity. Low HRV can be considered a transdiagnostic index for stress. It has also been found as a marker for consequent cardiovascular diseases, and generally worse health outcomes. Low HRV was associated with mental and behavioral impulses, and dysfunctional emotion regulation. Cattaneo et al. (2021) found that low HRV is associated with emotional dysregulation, worse cognitive performance, and transversal psychopathological conditions. In contrast, high HRV was associated with better executive function and emotion regulation supporting optimal functioning, good health, and appropriate activation of rational thinking of the frontal cortex. Cattaneo et al. (2021) discussed the importance of the vagus nerve as it supports bidirectional communication between the heart and the brain, especially during emotional reactions. They conclude that HRV is part of a complex system that incorporates and influences complex neurophysiological mechanisms, adaptive functions, and above all, it is a bidirectional system between central elements and peripheral/autonomic elements (heart and brain).

Role of positive emotions

A strategy to promote HRV regulation is to practice positive emotions such as gratitude, feeling love, and evoking sensations of joy and happiness. Some add a practice of prayer, uplifting instrumental music, chanting, or singing. Shifting to a positive emotional state can increase oxytocin which lowers stress hormones, which reduces blood pressure, improves mood, and increases tolerance for pain (Ong et al., 2011). Positive emotions may also contribute to the delay of the onset of disease and extend healthy functioning in later life. Positive emotion has been associated with reduced exposure to acute health conditions including incident stroke, myocardial infarction, and rehospitalization for coronary problems (Pressman & Cohen, 2005). Ong et al. (2011) describe several pathways for this association through improved behaviors, better sleep, better immune functioning, less reactivity to stressors, and reduced exposure to stressful health conditions.

Ricard et al. (2014) found that a positive outlook on life has been associated with lower blood pressure, reduced cardiovascular risk, better weight control, healthy blood sugar levels, and increased longevity. They link physical health such as neuronal health and neural functioning, cardiovascular health, immune function, and endocrine physiology to how people respond to stress. Those who may be more resilient to stress are better able to hold on to positive emotions such as people who practice stress reduction or meditation.

Meditation practices

Mindfulness meditation

There are a variety of meditation practices that may assist with improving health. A popular approach is mindfulness which is the practice of being present and aware. Jon Kabat-Zinn popularized mindfulness to Western society with his seminal psoriasis study (Kabat-Zinn et al., 1998). In this study, patients with moderate to severe psoriasis were treated with ultraviolet phototherapy (UVB) or photochemotherapy (PUVA). Half also had engaged in a mindfulness-based stress reduction intervention guided by audiotaped instructions during the light treatments. Those with mindfulness had significantly more rapid clearing than those without mindfulness. The practice of mindfulness is focusing on being present (perhaps by focusing on the breath or counting), acknowledging and noticing one's experience without judgment. Mindfulness teaches people how to be present. As a result, it slows racing thoughts, helps people release or disengage from negative thinking, and calms the nervous system by focusing on the here and now.

In mindfulness awareness, people are instructed to simply notice their experience without trying to change it, judge it, resist it, release it, or do anything about it. Just notice it and experience it. If clients notice their thoughts are going into a memory from the past, or worry about the future, or are distracted by other intrusive thoughts such as thinking about what one is going to do after meditating, they are guided to gently redirect their thoughts to simply observing and experiencing this moment. Breathing and just being, allowing oneself to be present in this moment, focusing on this breath.

Some helpful metaphors are the following: "Feelings are like waves; they come and they go." "Feelings are like clouds; watch them pass by in the sky." With each of these phrases, instruct clients to imagine their thoughts and feelings coming and going "like a wave" or "like a cloud" and to observe them without getting caught up in them. It is practiced by noticing and sensing what one is experiencing right now.

I offer another metaphor which is watching a train go by without getting on-board. The train is a line of thinking. Notice it, and let it pass. If you get on-board the train, it will take you far away to a distant place, other than right here. Instead, recognize it, notice it, and let it pass.

Integrative restoration

Richard Miller developed integrative restoration (iREST) adapted from the yoga Nidra tradition. The practice consists of moving through layers of awareness after setting one's intention, identifying one's heart's desire, and connecting with an inner place of ease. Awareness is brought to the body via a body scan, the breath, thoughts, feelings, and joy. Participants are guided to consider opposites (one side then the other side) and then to make room to hold the duality at the same time. This helps to diffuse from a particular thought or feeling and lays a foundation for non-duality, or non-separation.

Research is accumulating showing consistent evidence of reduced symptoms. Pence et al. (2014) conducted a small study with women veterans who experienced military sexual trauma. After 19 (90-minute) sessions they reported decreases in symptoms of posttraumatic stress disorder, negative thoughts of self-blame, and depression. Participants also offered verbal reports of decreased body tension, improved quality of sleep, improved ability to handle intrusive thoughts, improved ability to manage stress, and an increased feeling of joy.

Loving kindness meditation

Loving kindness meditation consists of focusing and saying positive statements with the intention of sending well-wishes for oneself and others. This practice promotes goodwill towards others and can improve stress reduction, increase a sense of social connectedness, and bring calm to one's nervous system. Kearney et al. (2013) conducted a study with veterans who had PTSD and found that engaging in deep, meaningful compassion and self-love meditations reduced trauma and flashback episodes. In a randomized controlled study, groups that received loving-kindness meditation scripts during their sessions could resume work sooner than participants who received other forms of guided instructions (Kearney et al., 2013). Research has also found that loving kindness meditation increases vagal tone as measured by heart rate variability.

Loving kindness is practiced by focusing, and repeating phrases with heartfelt intention for oneself, others, and the world. Example phrases could be: *May I be happy. May I be safe. May I be healthy. May I be at peace.* Say each phrase out loud, pause, and repeat each one three times, then go to the next phrase. Then, with someone in mind repeat, *May you be happy. May you be safe. May you be healthy. May you be at peace.* Repeating each phrase out loud three times. Finally, say each phrase for the world, *May the world be happy, May the world be safe, May the world be healthy, May the world be at peace.*

Alternatively, end the meditation with: *May you and I be happy. May you and I be safe. May you and I be healthy. May you and I be at peace.*

This is something that can be sandwiched between the signal and cleansing breath. Perhaps include a few minutes of mindfulness awareness before or after the phrases.

With loving-kindness meditation comes a profound spiritual transformation and the urge to reflect on our positive emotions (Kabat-Zinn, 1990).

Coping skills for managing emotions and trauma symptoms

Breathing and grounding exercises

Slow deep breathing

HRV can improve with slow deep breathing. Slow deep breathing is an easy skill to learn and practice with tangible effects on regulation and to improve optimal functioning. This can be used for an in-the-moment shift and with practice it can also reset one's resting baseline. For example, taking a few minutes every morning and evening to sit quietly and practice slow deep breathing helps to retrain the nervous system. Seppälä et al. (2014) found that Sudarshan kriya yoga a form of controlled breathing meditation showed significant decreases on hyperarousal startle response, re-experiencing symptoms, and generalized anxiety in a sample of U.S. male veterans of the Iraq or Afghanistan War compared to a wait-list control group. Findings were sustained one year later.

Grounding

A single deep exhale, releasing through the shoulders, dropping down into the belly, is truly the quickest and easiest way to reset, and calm. Bringing one's awareness through the feet, grounding by wiggling the toes and pressing into the earth, enhances the calm. A third layer is lifting arms with the inhale, matching movement with breath, and lowering with the exhale completes this grounding exercise. This is helpful for anxiety, dissociation, or not feeling present in one's mind or body.

Other grounding techniques include engaging the senses:

- *Sight*: Gazing by turning one's head to left and right, scanning the room, orienting to the room
- *Sound*: Listen to the sounds around you, perhaps closing your eyes
- *Smell*: Smell the air or a pleasant scent (e.g., from a candle or aromatherapy oil); scent goes to the midbrain and can have an immediate effect on mood

- *Touch*: Holding a smooth rock, soft blanket, or other object to engage physical sensation of touch
- *Taste*: Sucking on a mint can help ground to the here and now

In addition, being aware of food and drink can impact grounding. Caffeine and sugar can mimic symptoms of anxiety and dysregulation. Alcohol can magnify depression or anger. In contrast, protein can help people feel more grounded and at ease in their bodies. Water can also help with physical and emotional detoxification. An overall balanced diet with good hydration can assist with grounding. Nonetheless, when people feel emotionally dysregulated, they may reach for processed or sugary food or drink, alcohol, or other substances for comfort or distraction, only to exacerbate their dysregulation. Diet and substance use is something to address with clients. One way to describe this is stacking the cards in one's favor, and choosing behaviors that will support their well-being. In contrast, the choice to use food, drink, or other substances in times of stress, is like driving your car with the emergency-brake on. It goes against your goals, it makes it difficult, in some cases impossible to move forward.

The power of smell

Further discussion of smell is worthwhile given its powerful and immediate effect for grounding. Smell travels through the nose via the cranial nerve to the olfactory bulb which is located in the limbic system, where emotions are processed in the brain. The limbic system is also where the amygdala resides, which plays a role in regulating emotional memories and activating the fight/flight/freeze response. The olfactory system also relates to the part of the brain called the hippocampus which is critical in developing memories. Because the olfactory bulb can influence both the amygdala and the hippocampus, smell can have a powerful effect on either recalling or interrupting emotional memory. Smell can be used to help ground oneself after anxiety, panic, or a nightmare. Smell goes directly to the emotional center of the brain not through the thinking part of the brain. This is particularly helpful because the thinking part may be activated with negative thoughts and may not be able to shift very quickly. But a smell works almost instantaneously, regardless of what one is thinking about.

Signal breath

The signal breath is helpful to address anger, frustration, or fear. It is called a signal breath because like a traffic signal, it helps you slow down, stop, and then move forward in a more relaxed frame of mind. It is based on two principles: 1) you can't be relaxed and tense at the same time, and 2) everything is connected... so, if you relax your mind, then you also relax your body, and if you relax your body, then you relax your mind. It is practiced like this: *"Take in a deep breath inhaling through your nose into your diaphragm. Hold it at the top of the breath, for several seconds (up to 5 if that's comfortable for you). Then, let it out slowly through your mouth. As you exhale, imagine all of the tension leaving your body."*

Cleansing breath

The cleansing breath is easy and effective. It is practiced like this: *"Take a deep breath in through the nose and let it out with a heavy sigh."* The breath is not held during this exercise. It is designed to cleanse away tension in the body. It can be used anywhere or anytime when you want a quick release of tension. Try this without the sigh and then with the sigh to feel the difference.

Relaxation sandwich

The relaxation sandwich (Katz, 2014) is a way to begin and end a relaxation session. Start with 2–3 signal breaths, then a single or series of relaxation exercises, and end with 1–2 cleansing breaths. The two breaths are like the bread and any other exercise is the filling of the sandwich. For example, a relaxation sandwich may be two signal breaths, three minutes of mindful awareness, and two cleansing breaths.

Calming hand positions

There are several calming hand positions that may be used on their own or in conjunction with deep breathing or meditation. The hand poses bring balance, calming, focus, and soothing.

Hand pose #1: Prayer position. Place palms of hands together. Hold hands midway to the chest (at the heart), thumbs to the chest, fingers spread out so the pinky fingers point outward. Hold the pose… breathing. This can be done with eyes open or closed.

Hand pose #2: Heart and belly. Start this pose by rubbing hands together, and then placing right hand on the chest, and left hand on the belly (palms facing towards the body). Feel the warmth of the hands going into the body. This is particularly good for bringing comfort (e.g., to soothe grief, anxiety or worry). It is calming and easily coupled with mindfulness, deep breathing, or listening to comforting music. Support elbows with pillows if holding for extended time.

Hand pose #3: Neck and forehead. Start this pose by rubbing hands together, and then placing right hand on the forehead, and left hand at the back of the neck (at the base of the head) with palms facing towards the head. Feel the warmth and soothing nature of this pose. This is particularly good for headaches, and racing thoughts.

Hand pose #4: Shoulder hug. Extend both arms in front, palms facing together. Place right palm on left shoulder and left palm on right shoulder. This mimics the sensation of receiving a hug. It is comforting and reassuring which is particularly helpful after deep transformative work like imagery reprocessing.

COPE (cleansing breath, observation, positive self-talk, explanation)

A simple effective strategy is COPE (Katz, 2005, 2014) C stands for Cleansing breath, O stands for Observation, P stands for Positive self-talk, and E stands for Explanation. COPE may be useful for calming, and putting anxiety into perspective. The feeling will pass like water flowing through a hose.

Cleansing breath. "*A cleansing breath is a deep inhale through the nose and exhale with a sigh.*" Because people who are anxious tend to hold their breath, it is useful to work on fully exhaling the breath, thereby releasing tension and facilitating breathing.

Observation. "*There are two things to observe. First observe the environment to reassure yourself that there is no actual danger in the present moment. Next observe the fight, flight, and freeze reaction of anxiety that is occurring in your body. Recognize that you are having normal symptoms of anxiety such as increased heart rate, sweating, light-headedness, and tight muscles.*"

Positive self-talk. "*Tell yourself positive and comforting statements. Reassure yourself that you're okay, this will pass, breathe, you're safe, etc. What can you say to yourself that will make you feel better when this happens?*"

Explanation. "*Remind yourself that this is only a trauma trigger (something in the present that reminds me of the past, but is not actually dangerous).*" Having a label to understand what is going on will lessen the intensity of the experience. Imagine the difference between telling yourself statements such as "*What is happening to me? I might be having a heart attack! Everyone is staring at me!*" These are typical thoughts that people have when they are triggered. However, notice how much calmer you would feel if you told yourself something like this: "*I'm okay, I know what this is… It's a trigger of anxiety and it will pass in a couple of minutes. I'm having a normal fight or flight response to a perception of threat but because there is no danger, it is safe to calm down. I'm going to just watch myself have this experience and know it will pass as I continue to take slow deep breaths, exhaling completely.*"

Cleansing breath: Inhale through the nose, exhale with a sigh. Take several slow, deep, breaths, exhaling completely

Observation: Realize there is no danger, observe sensations and thoughts come and go
Positive self-talk: "I'm okay, and this will pass"
Explanation: "This is an intrusive thought. This is just a normal response to a trigger"

Positive focal point

A positive focal point helps people stay present, disrupts repetitive negative thinking, and gives them a specific focus. This is very helpful when retraining the mind from focusing on the past and staying present. This is also helpful with intrusive negative thoughts. A positive focal point can be an image, a color, a song, prayer, a phrase, smell, or anything that the client chooses as a positive place to rest their mind, provide reassurance or comfort.

A safe place imagery

In this exercise, clients are instructed to use visualization to imagine a place that is safe, comforting, and pleasant. Some clients prefer to create a fantasy place while others prefer to recall a specific memory. The imagery may or may not include other people. If clients do not have a specific memory, then the therapist can suggest a nature scene such as on the beach, by a tropical waterfall, or in the mountains. Ask what the client prefers and then fill in the details of the scene including colors, sounds, smells, and textures. Anchor a positive feeling associated with the scene. For example, a therapist might say, *"Imagine that you feel very relaxed and whenever you imagine this beautiful place you feel happy, safe, comfortable, and calm."*

Snapshot

A positive focal point or safe place image can be a snapshot or a quick image that is practiced to disrupt something negative. The following are examples of snapshots chosen by various clients: an image of a sunflower, the color green, driving with the window down, a certain prayer, playing ball with my grandson, my dogs, and lyrics from a favorite song. With practice this is an effective tool to refocus one's mind.

Washing machine metaphor

The washing machine metaphor (Katz, 2014) helps people observe their experience of having a trigger, or bout of anxiety without getting caught up in it. Like COPE, it helps reduce the intensity and duration of the upset.

"Imagine being inside a washing machine during a wash cycle. You and the clothes, soap, and water are getting tossed about. You are in it, so you can't see that there is a beginning or end to it. Just chaos out of your control, and all you can do is survive. This is what it is like when you have trauma symptoms. Life is a series of tumble and spin cycles."

"Now step out of the washing machine. You can see the clothes and soap and water spinning around. It may be chaos in there, but you can watch it without getting caught up in it. You can see that it is a temporary cycle, with a beginning and end, and the clothes are going to be fine." This is using the observer vantage point to notice oneself going through an emotional reaction or symptom of trauma such as a trauma trigger, nightmare, panic attack, or other bout of upset, and watch it pass.

Healthy distraction

It is helpful to have a list of healthy distractions to give your mind a chance to calm and reset. Once in a calmer state, it is easier to think and engage the rational mind for healthy choices and responses.

Here are some examples:

• Go for a walk
• Watch an uplifting movie
• Call a friend
• Take a drive
• Listen to music
• Read a book or magazine

Anger and resentment

Most of the skills discussed thus far, have been focused on reducing anxiety-types of reactions. However, anger and resentment are particularly insidious and can keep people stuck in a state of affect dysregulation. Anger can be both a symptom and cause of affect dysregulation, possibly leading to serious consequences to self and others. Unlike the other strategies that focus on calming the nervous system (e.g., deep breathing), addressing chronic anger or resentment requires a cognitive component (which will be discussed further in Chapter 10). People usually feel justified in their anger. For many, the root of anger is injustice. Something was gravely wrong, unfair, or violated someone or something in a wholly unacceptable way. Anger may be appropriate. There *was* a wrong, an injustice, and it was not fair. For some, any trigger brings up an automatic reaction of anger. Calming strategies in and of itself does not alter the reasoning or justification for why they are angry.

As a result, anger interferes with peace, well-being, relationships, and health. It can be used to justify substance abuse or acting out against others, because someone is angry. And anger can feed on itself, derailing someone's logical thinking and/or reinforce negative, categorical (all or nothing), grandiose, and self-centered thinking. It can also lead to other gross logical distortions (taking one comment to mean a host of things that may not be true at all). Anger can reinforce distrust, fear, paranoia, leading to heightened anxiety and depression.

Rage, a form of outwardly expressed anger, can be loud, unpredictable, and potentially dangerous. Resentment, a form of chronic quiet anger, can linger like smoldering coals left behind when the fire is gone. Resentments can build when there is no restitution, no apology, no amends. The injustice sits and festers at the bottom of one's stomach.

It's a conundrum: anger can be both justified and can derail one's health and well-being.

People can get stuck ruminating about their own experiences of injustice such as "This was taken from me." Maybe so. Things might have been better, or maybe not. We cannot assume another path would have been a better path.

Being stuck in anger and resentments from the past interferes with joy and building a better future.

When clients are ready to release their anger (after doing the work of considering context and other strategies such as *Poetic Justice* presented in Chapter 10), it can be helpful to discuss being in the here and now. *"You cannot change the past, but what are you going to do now to move your life in a better direction? You can still meet people, earn money, improve your health, expand your consciousness, help others, and do something productive and meaningful. Activities such as these may bring joy and fulfillment to yourself and others. You cannot change or undo the past. But you can gather up your resources and forge ahead."*

A meditation for clients to release anger

"I know and you know what happened was wrong. I release myself from thinking about what you did. I will let that be yours to contend with. I release myself from any energetic ties to you, I wipe my hands, and free myself from you and the past." (Imagery: imaging energetic threads connecting you to the past or past perpetrator. Imagine cutting the strings, like thin rubber bands springing free, releasing oneself, feeling light, and relieved.)

This is what Antonio (this chapter's case example) did to release himself from intrusive thoughts about his past. He had to release his chronic negative thoughts of anger and injustice. He worked on disengaging his connection with what happened in his past.

Script for resetting and regulating one's nervous system

"Find a comfortable place to sit or lie down, with your body feeling supported. Drop into a place of ease. Bring your attention to feeling present in your body. Use a calming hand position, or let your hands rest comfortably in your lap. You can start with a signal breath, a deep breath in through the nose, hold it at the top for 5 seconds, and then exhale through the mouth. Next bring your focus to your breath. Practice slow deep breathing, extending the inhale for about 5 seconds and the exhale for about 5 seconds. Slow even breaths. Staying present... and breathing. If you'd like, think of your positive focal point or positive image to help you feel a positive emotion, something that makes you feel good like gratitude or love... something that makes you feel happy. Think of an image or something that makes you smile (a pet, loved ones, being at the beach, or even a large hot fudge sundae!). ... hold on to that feeling, growing it in your body, while letting the image fade away. Allow yourself to exhale completely, releasing any tension in your body. Maybe your shoulders or chest release a bit more. Keep your focus on being present and continue slow deep breathing. If a thought comes up, just let it pass by like a cloud passing in the sky. Enjoying this moment, this breath. And when you are ready, take in a deep breath and release with a sigh. And again, big breath in... stretching... and exhale with a sigh. Inhale opening to life, and exhale releasing all that no longer serves you."

(See Appendix B for an extended version.)

Chapter summary

Emotion regulation is the foundation for managing triggers. It also helps return to higher cortical thinking, which improves the ability to consider consequences and alternatives, engage in problem-solving, improve communication, and have empathy for others. Several strategies, exercises and metaphors were presented for grounding, breathing, and calming.

Coping skills for managing emotions and trauma symptoms

Grounding
Signal and cleansing breaths
Calming hand poses
COPE
Positive focal point
Washing machine metaphor
Healthy distraction
Meditation for releasing anger and resentment
Script for resetting and regulating one's nervous system

Chapter 7

Experiential discovery

This chapter presents strategies for exploring and identifying experiential holograms, particularly interpersonal experiential holograms, by utilizing associations activated by the experiential system. Various strategies are presented such as experiential focusing, making a time-line of significant events and relationships, and journaling.

Case example: "Loveable after all"

I met Cassie an outgoing trans-woman. We instantly had a good rapport. She had completed a series of seminar courses on self-improvement and was feeling motivated. However, she was coming to see me for something else. She was very articulate and seemed to choose her words carefully and deliberately. She understood concepts quickly but emotionally, she was still stuck. We identified her fear around expressing her feelings and the need to be in control. I felt her exhale as if finally, someone understood her pain. By the end of the first session, she stated that she knew this therapy would be helpful for her.

In the next session, she discussed her pain of wanting to stay in her current relationship but was struggling to live with a man that was emotionally withholding. She had been living with him and his son for the past six months. Throughout their relationship, he maintained a special friendship with another woman and made it clear that he would not give her up. He would have private weekend meetings with this friend. He claimed it was not about sex but he did spend the night with her on these weekends. She stated she was frustrated with his inability to commit to her.

The third week she called in tears. Through her tears she stated she was just fired from her job and her boyfriend asked her to move out of the house. She continued to cry and asked for an earlier session. The following is an account of that session.

Cassie came into the session in tears. She stated she felt so bad she just wanted to die. She said that she was fired from her job because they thought

DOI: 10.4324/9781003223429-9

she was leaking information to their competitor. She said they thought it was her because she was taking work home with her. She admitted that she was taking the work home so she could complete it. She was fired anyway and the night before her boyfriend said their relationship "wasn't working out" and she needed to move out.

I asked her to tell me what makes these things so upsetting to her. She looked at me like "Wasn't it obvious?" I said it would be helpful if she could articulate it. I gave her a prompt to complete: "I'm upset because..." and I began to take notes. She said, "I'm upset because I'm afraid of losing control, I'm afraid of not having a job, I don't know what's going to happen and where I'm going to live and how I'm going to pay for the bills." "And this is upsetting to me because..." I encouraged. "This is upsetting to me because I feel insecure and vulnerable. I feel like giving up. I can never make our relationship work if I move out." "And this is upsetting because..." "This is upsetting because I didn't want it to work out this way. I'm all alone again. I feel so hurt and unwanted. I didn't even defend myself, I just said, ok and left. It's my fault for not trying harder." "And this makes you feel...?" I gently continued. "Like I'm completely rejected and unlovable!"

I listened to this list and circled the words hurt, unwanted, rejected, and unlovable. These were the words of her experiential system and I hypothesized the doorway to her experiential hologram. (*Note*: "the trying harder," "afraid of losing control/staying in control," "I can make it work" are compensating strategies.) I told her I thought what was really upsetting to her was being rejected and feeling hurt, unwanted, and unlovable. She nodded and confirmed that that was exactly how she felt.

I asked if she remembers the first time she experienced these feelings. Because she was currently experiencing these emotions, it should facilitate the recall of other incidents of similar feelings. This is consistent with state-dependent learning. To whatever incident she would remember I would typically ask if there was something earlier. This is an attempt to get to the initial source of the core hologram. We discussed the prompts, "What am I feeling?" and "Have I felt this way before?" She closed her eyes, placed her hands over her heart and focused. She asked herself, "What am I feeling?" She said, "unlovable." "Have I felt this way before?" She said she felt this way in grammar school when nobody played with her at recess. She wanted to hang out with the girls but they didn't want her. After a moment and an empathic, "hmm," I asked, "Something before that?" She breathed, still with hands on her heart, and said, "the first time I felt rejected was in my mother's womb."

She stated she always had a feeling that her mother didn't want her. Her mother also confirmed that she was in pain when she was pregnant. She stated her father never wanted her either. As a child she remembered feeling a mixture of hurt and defiance. She stated, "You don't want me? That's too bad I'm here anyway!" (That defiance has served her well in owning herself and claiming herself as a woman.)

She stated that it was her grandmother who gave her warmth and attention. She remembers being raised by her grandmother while her mother went to work. When her grandmother died, she experienced a deep sense of loss. We spent the rest of the session mapping her pattern of a rejection hologram by completing a pot on the stove template.

She described her experience from a child's perspective and I wondered what else was going on. In other words, we were ready to explore the context of the situation. I asked her to tell me about her mother (i.e., how old was she, what was going on during the time she was pregnant, etc.). She stated her mother was 19 years old, pregnant with her, and in the middle of getting a divorce. I asked her what she thought her mother was feeling at the time of pregnancy and during her early childhood. Cassie said, "Oh, she was confused and overwhelmed. Even if she was in emotional pain, she would just focus on survival, mustering up all her strength and avoiding her feelings." She said she was frustrated by this because she would want to talk about her feelings and her mother would say, "feelings don't pay the bills." (Another example of her feeling rejected/unloved by her mother.) Cassie said she saw that she had become just like her mother—focusing on survival and avoiding her feelings.

We paused at this point in the session for Cassie to feel what it was really like for her mother. I told her to imagine herself as a 19-year-old in the same situation and how truly difficult that must have been for her. Next, I began to inquire about her initial feelings of being unwanted, rejected, and unlovable. I again asked her to focus on what it would be like to be pregnant if you weren't sure that you could provide a stable, comfortable future for your child. Cassie looked up and said her mother thought about having an abortion but she didn't. Her father pressured her to do it, but her mother said no. "Nineteen years old, getting a divorce, and being pregnant, she must have been really worried about being a good mother, and a good provider for me..." Cassie started to cry.

I reinforced, "So you are saying your mother chose to have you, and provided for you the best she could. Why do you think so?" "Because she loved me?" "Sounds like she loved you *very much*." Cassie nodded her head and continued to cry. I said, "You have been living from the reality that you are unlovable, but that is not true! Both your mother and grandmother loved you. You are and have always been loved." Cassie said, "I get that. I never thought about it before. She did choose to have me... and take care of me." We breathed together, relishing in her new version of reality. She stated, "I feel like I am in a different world. It's like I integrated something so I can see the positive and negative at the same time."

She said she realized that her initial upset about the job and boyfriend were catalysts for a deeper healing.

The next week she stated she felt great and she couldn't remember ever feeling so good. She said it was difficult to describe, but it felt like all of her cells that were holding on to her old beliefs were now recalibrating. The next few sessions were aimed at integrating this new version of reality. We confronted some behavioral patterns that set herself up for feeling rejected. She loved the imagery reprocessing exercises to provide reassurance, comfort, and love to her younger self. She said, "I am good enough, and loved enough just the way I am."

She managed to find a new job and an apartment of her own. She had a breakthrough with her boyfriend as well. He told her that he is committed to being an important friend to her. Just because he could not handle being in a committed romantic relationship (with anyone) didn't negate his feelings towards her. Thus, she truly understood that she can be loveable even if someone had interfering issues (i.e., her mother and boyfriend). Those were their issues, and did not define her. This was a particularly powerful insight to realize other people's reactions are reflections of their own issues. This frees her from personalizing their issues.

How does one identify interpersonal experiential holograms?

In this case example, Cassie used associations to link her current feelings to experiences in her past. She was able to quickly connect to her feelings of being rejected and unlovable, and was very aware of how this was a theme from the beginning of her life. This is an experiential discovery process where clients are asked to focus on their feelings, associations, memories, and images. Cassie closed her eyes and instinctively placed her hands on her heart. She was relaxed, focusing on her experience, and letting her feelings guide her to her memories.

Emotions create a super-highway to facilitate recall of emotional memories which share similar emotional themes. This is based on CET theory of associations, experiential awareness, and communicating with the experiential system. As stated previously, the metaphor of a string of holiday lights helps explain how the string is the emotion, and the bulbs are various experiences (memories) that align with that emotion. Once the string is plugged in (activated) then related memories light up for easy retrieval.

Notice experiential discovery was used twice in this example first to find her core violation of rejection and her personal belief that she is unlovable, and again, when mentalizing about her mother at age 19. Since Cassie was in her thirties, she was able to imagine what that must have been like for her mother from a different vantage point rather than from being a child. This helped her understand her mother and herself in a new way.

Gene Gendlin, Ph.D. was an experiential psychologist who developed the technique called *focusing*. On his website for the International Focusing Institute, he explained that focusing is a form of "felt-sensing," where the body is a guide to self-knowledge and healing. Similarly, holographic reprocessing gathers information in the experiential system by bringing awareness to internal cues, such as feelings and bodily sensations and by asking a series of feeling-oriented questions. This could be asking oneself, "What am I feeling?" or a therapist might ask, "Where is the feeling in your body?" "Have you felt this way before?" Gendlin might ask, "What does the problem feel like? What word describes the feelings that seem to move the body forward?" Correctly identifying the feeling associated with a problem leads to a physical easing and a felt release.

To gain insight, clients may be asked to list feelings, describe a feeling, or focus on where they might feel a feeling in their body. Gendlin's website (http://focusing.org, pp. 135–137) states:

> Once a felt sense has come into focus (meaning it is more present, clear, and stable) one can move to the step Gendlin calls "asking." Simple questions like "What are you worried about?" or "What do you need?" ... Often (not always) if one waits patiently and gently, the felt sense will answer with an unexpected insight, an "Aha!" moment, along with a body sense of release or opening (often referred to as a "shift"). Something held deep inside has come unstuck, providing a new sense of direction and fresh energy to undertake it.

In both focusing and holographic reprocessing, clients may be taught how to scan their bodies for physical tension using a body scan, and are also taught the author's technique of the emotional scan, where clients scan the areas of tension in the body and identify associated emotions in each area of tension (Katz, 2001). After the tension and related emotions are identified, the client is asked to associate them with images, events, and memories.

The discovery process is an important and delicate phase in this therapy. It requires clients to open up parts of themselves which may feel particularly uncomfortable or vulnerable. The therapist needs to be sensitive to clients' experiences and reinforce that they can rely on their foundation of coping skills. As mentioned earlier, sometimes the process itself triggers an unfolding of associations in-between sessions. Clients may revert to old self-destructive coping strategies or may complain of increased symptoms. Therefore, this process should not be rushed.

Some clients may associate feelings to events that they have never spoken about or realized before. If this is the case, then the therapist and client may need to discuss how they want to address this. A supportive therapeutic alliance, reassurance, and encouragement can help. It's also appropriate to retreat and wait, maybe taking a cleansing breath, or just observe the experience to help clients stay present without triggering or avoiding content. Some clients may prefer to write about the incident before talking about it in therapy.

On the other hand, many clients report a sudden "ah-ha" or awareness, and feel a sense of relief as if finally, they connected to something that helps explain their life.

Techniques for experiential discovery

Connect with the experience

The first step is for the client to connect with their current emotions. It is not sufficient to intellectualize the feelings but rather important to feel them because it opens the channels for association. Therapists can ask clients where in the body they feel the feeling. This helps bring focus to the sensations in the body.

Label the feeling

To help clients articulate exactly what they are feeling, therapists can ask them to list everything they are feeling. If a client is having difficulty generating words, the therapist can help by listing several feelings and then asking if any resonate. When a particularly strong or accurate feeling is articulated, the client will have a felt-sense or experiential confirmation. Gendlin described that the body moves forward as a felt confirmation (Gendlin, 1996).

Free association following the feeling

Therapists can ask when the client has felt this feeling before and wait for memories, images, or other associations to arise. They can then discuss the association and listen to the aspects that connect to a broader theme in the client's life (Katz, 2001). Then we discuss what about the experience is upsetting. How does it make the person feel? What remains emotionally unresolved, conflicted, or is cause for distress? What aspects are incongruent with clients' assumptions about themselves, others, and the world? There are a variety of issues that may need to be addressed such as loss of power, self-blame, betrayal, loss of self-esteem. The discovery process finds out the specific associations and meanings for each person.

Example inquiry:

What am I feeling?
What else am I feeling?
And how does that feel in the body?
Anything else?
Is this the root feeling? (Does it move the body forward?)
Have I felt his way before?
This feeling reminds me of...

Example inquiry:

I'm upset because...
And this is upsetting because...
It makes me feel...
What else do I feel?

What if clients have difficulty accessing feelings?

Some clients may not be able to access or label their feelings. Others may feel self-conscious in front of their therapist. Several alternative strategies may be used. One is creating a time-line of events. Clients list their significant life events or relationships in chronological order. Dynamics of the events or relationships are discussed. Therapists and clients can reflect on the information to identify repeating patterns or themes among the noted events. The themes are working hypotheses for identifying the client's experiential hologram. As a follow-up they can explore if the theme has been present in other situations such as on a job, or with other people not already mentioned.

Clients can journal to further explore the themes in their lives. They can journal about their nightmares and dreams, or types of intrusive thoughts/daydreams, or relationship patterns. Some journal prompts can be activating, so these should be implemented with caution such as the prompt, "I'm angry because... I'm also angry because.... And this makes me angry because... until getting to the core issue of the anger." Good clinical judgment should be exercised.

The following are some tools to help people identify themes in their relationships and common patterns that may reveal the components of their experiential hologram. The therapist may ask these questions or clients may answer the questions on the client-version handout available in Appendix C. Included in this appendix is the *Interpersonal Experiential Hologram Inventory (IEHI)* to help clients identify themes and components of their experiential hologram.

The discovery process, in general, is designed to be collaborative between therapists and clients. Therapists are encouraged to stay with the spirit of discovery until both therapist and client agree that the description of the experiential hologram resonates on an experiential level, or in other words, "it feels right."

Questions for discovering interpersonal experiential holograms (adapted from Holographic Reprocessing, Katz, 2005)

1   What does the client find initially attractive in someone? Or motivates their interaction?
2   What disappoints the client about the other person?
     (This reveals some of the negative qualities of the other person. They expected them to be one way but they turned out to be another way. The therapist must use skill to distinguish between a general negative event and specifically what is emotionally violating about that relationship.)
3   How does the client feel after the relationship is over or after the relationship has been going on for a while?
     (This question helps to articulate client's relationship experiences. How were they treated and how did that feel?)
4   What does the client think about themselves being in this relationship or after it is over?
     (This question helps identify personal truths or thoughts about oneself.)
5   How does the client respond to those feelings?
     (This reveals the clients avoidant and compensating strategies. The therapist can ask this question and explore a variety of strategies. The therapist might ask, "What else do you do when you feel this way?")
6   How does the client feel in between relationships?
     (This helps reveal the linger feelings or residual emotional states between cycles of the hologram.)

Brief tool for Identifying Interpersonal holograms

The following is a journaling exercise. The therapist explains the rationale of the exercise: to help identify relationship patterns. Ultimately, for the purpose to free themselves from having to continue to repeat the same relationship dynamics. This should be presented as a learning opportunity but approached with compassion. This is not about blame, but rather it is about awareness. These exercises may help bring forward several themes. There are several components to an interpersonal experimental hologram discussed in detail in the next chapter.

Instructions: "The following questions are designed to help you think about the relationships in your life. There are no right or wrong answers—

just do the best you can to answer the questions. Do not overthink each question but rather go with your automatic response."

- First make a list of several relationships you have had.
- What qualities were attractive to you in these relationships?
- After you were involved in the relationship, what qualities did they have that disappointed you?
- How did you feel at the end of these relationships or after an extended time?

Connecting to your childhood or formative relationships, did you feel similar emotions? Was this feeling similar perhaps, to how you felt with a parent or caregiver? Was it similar to what you observed in your parents' relationship? What do you think contributed to this feeling? How about during other times of your life?

Experiential discovery is about reflecting, listening, and exploring common themes. The inquiry could be about relationships but also could be inclusive of significant life events as a source to reveal unresolved issues. For example, Sandra had a recent suicide attempt where she was drinking and then jumped out of a window. She noted the emotions and mindset that precipitated the event. She was not sure why she did it. With experiential discovery, she associated her feelings with an experience she had with her grandfather. She was five years old. He lured her to his room with promises of candy and forced her to engage in a sexual act. She had a spontaneous recovered memory that at the time of the abuse, she was focusing on jumping out of the window to escape. Once recalled, her adult behavior made sense to her in a new way. When she felt trapped, she wanted to jump out of a window.

Common mistakes when engaging in experiential discovery

As discussed in Katz (2005), there could be several common mistakes that therapists might make when they are first learning experiential discovery. 1) They may not be engaging the client's experiential system which activates the system of associations. 2) They may have difficulty identifying a client's feelings. 3) They may not take the time to go deep enough to do an adequate discovery about other feelings to find the one that moves the body forward. 4) They may not take the time to fully explore the associations to uncover client core violations and associated emotional and behavioral responses.

In an example presented in Katz (2005), a trainee reported that his client's issue is that she felt her friend was selfish. Further inquiry led to the client feeling hatred, and finally they concluded that she felt her friend was a jerk. This was an attempt at experiential discovery but labeling the friend a jerk did not lead to insight or moving the body forward. The first issue is the declaration that the client felt her friend was selfish is not a feeling. It is a thought, more specifically, a judgment about her friend. Using the word feeling does not necessarily mean it is a feeling. This is important as experiential discovery is predicated on connecting with feelings to access the experiential system. There may be an implication of a feeling such as hurt, disappointment, or anger and this is what should have been explored. Nonetheless, they did get to a feeling of hatred. This is a strong feeling which has the potential for fruitful associations and discovery. Perhaps hatred was related to anger, then hurt, and then to a host of other feelings such as jealousy, feeling betrayed, or neglected. This would have given a rich glimpse into the client's experiential system and could have opened up a discussion about relationships where she felt similar feelings. Unfortunately, the exploration process was halted prematurely.

For some, staying on a feeling level may be uncomfortable, for both clients and therapists. Therapists may have to confront their own feelings to be able to hold a space for ambiguity, negative affect, and witnessing and resonating with another's heart-felt pain. It may be more comfortable to distance from feelings, focus on intellectualization, or work on behaviors. And clients may willingly collude with avoiding experiential exploration. However, the gain for connecting with feelings, listening to what arises, and truly getting to the root issue that is repeated in someone's life can lead to deep transformational work.

Using the architecture blueprints metaphor, experiential discovery starts at one house (where a house = a relationship), examining the issues in one's current relationships. Then clients are asked if this issue was found in any other house that they built? If the same issue is present in several houses, we can deduce something is amiss on the underlying blueprint. The discovery process helps clients and therapists get to their relationship blueprint.

Memory loss

What if your client knows they were abused but has no specific memories? This could be significant memory loss from childhood or memory loss during events of trauma at any age. Because of the associative nature of the experiential mind, if there is a pattern (e.g., persistent issue), or personalization (e.g., beliefs about oneself), then these will be present at the current time. It is not necessary to remember the past in order to heal.

Holographic reprocessing is about releasing the past by helping people resolve what is keeping them stuck. It could be a persistent negative belief about themselves or others that is expressed in various relationships and circumstances in the present. In many cases, it's about letting go of responsibility for other people's behavior. With or without memories, nobody is responsible for their own abuse.

It is not necessary to remember details of abuse, in order to heal.

Chapter summary

This chapter presents various techniques to engage in experiential discovery or connecting with core issues related to one's experiential hologram. Using the associative properties of the experiential system, clients can access formative events. Emotional feelings and body sensations are the super highways to the experiential system to facilitate this discovery. The basic technique for experiential discovery is to connect with a current emotional experience, label the feeling, sense it in the body, and allow for associated images or memories to surface. Clients can journal by completing question prompts, or the Interpersonal Experiential Hologram Inventory (see Appendix C) to help identify patterns and related coping strategies.

Chapter 8

Interpersonal experiential holograms

Experiential holograms are patterns of re-enactments, formed from experiences of maltreatment and abuse, that reside in the experiential system, are projections from neural networks (the past), and appear to be real. This chapter explains the four main clusters of interpersonal experiential holograms, with examples for each. A guided inquiry process is presented to help identify holographic types. It also presents a template of the pot on a stove to map the six components of an interpersonal experiential hologram.

Four case examples of interpersonal experiential holograms

Amy has a neglect hologram

Amy was a sweet, caring, and soft-spoken woman in her mid-fifties. When she checked in to the clinic, she was always kind and thoughtful of others. She knew the names of all the staff at the front office, asked about their children, and brought them cookies to show her appreciation. One day there was a mix-up. Someone else came to the clinic thinking it was her time for an appointment, but she had come on the wrong day. Amy quickly said it was "ok," gave up her appointment time to the other client, and said she would call to reschedule. She left so it would not cause any issues. Amy was being treated for depression. She felt drained, exhausted, lonely, and wanted to lose weight.

Helen has a rejection hologram

Helen was enrolled in college. She came to the clinic seeking an evaluation for adult attention deficit hyperactivity disorder (ADHD). She said she wanted a letter to bring to her school to give her extra time for test taking due to anxiety and her inability to focus. She said when she sits down for a test, her mind goes blank, and that makes her panic. She starts to shake. She can't focus and has difficulty sitting in her seat. Helen was a high achiever, very self-critical, detail-oriented, and holds high expectations for herself. To

DOI: 10.4324/9781003223429-10

her, any grade less than an A is an F. She was worried about her grades, her future, and had a fear of complete failure.

Samuel has a betrayal hologram

Samuel was self-employed after being fired twice for angry outbursts and getting into fights with co-workers. He was seeking therapy because his wife served him divorce papers and a restraining order. She said she won't let him see his daughter unless he got therapy for his anger. Samuel said he doesn't trust anyone because everyone was a liar and a thief.

Olivia has an endangerment hologram

Olivia came to therapy because her boyfriend insisted that she gets help for her eating disorder. Olivia had a severe eating disorder (bulimia nervosa) with daily bouts of food binges followed by self-induced vomiting. She knew this was a problem and disclosed that her boyfriend didn't know how bad it really was. She hid food in her car, ate when he went out, and found ways to shield him from the full extent of her issue. She had high credit card debt from her spending, but the bill went to a post-office box so her boyfriend didn't see it. While sitting in therapy, she discretely ordered meals on her phone to eat after the session. She grew up in a strict family and it was important to live up to the high expectations of her parents, particularly her mother. When her older brother started sexually abusing her, she could not tell anyone. Her parents idolized her brother. She had to pretend everything was fine, while she was being criticized, shamed, and sexually abused. She avoided her family and dreaded the weekly phone call with her mother.

Common types of interpersonal experiential holograms

There are several types of emotional traumas or core violations that can be the driving force for people's interpersonal experiential holograms such as being neglected, rejected, betrayed, or endangered. These are not events such as "rape," or "being bullied." But rather, is the underlying emotionally painful part of the experience? When we discuss an event of sexual trauma, what about it remains emotionally haunting and deeply upsetting? Perhaps it was life-threatening, or maybe it was the deep hurt of a betrayal from a trusted friend. The same event can mean different things to different people.

Based on attachment theory, there are four elements of secure attachment: feeling loved, safe, and free to explore one's word (autonomy), and having healthy boundaries and limits. These elements are on a continuum. When good enough, these can lead to a secure attachment. When one or more is inadequate, it can lead to an insecure attachment. Examining these elements on a continuum in the chart shown in Figure 8.1, it shows patterns of lacking elements leaning towards one of the four quadrants, corresponds to one of four main interpersonal experiential hologram types.

Four interpersonal experiential holograms

Neglected = Feeling unloved + lack of boundaries/inattention
Rejected = Feeling unloved + critical, demanding, controlling
Betrayed = Feeling unsafe + lack of boundaries/inattention
Endangered = Feeling unsafe + critical, demanding, controlling

Neglect trauma

Neglect occurs when someone feels emotionally or physically ignored, not protected from harm, not listened to, believed, understood, not being nurtured or loved, and not being taken care of. Neglect may leave people feeling unworthy, invisible, and unimportant (e.g., their needs don't matter). In response to feeling unattended to, a common strategy is to connect with others by attending to others. This may include being helpful, caring, funny, sexy, overly responsible, or overly attentive to others. The implicit hope is that if they are attentive, then others will appreciate them, and attend to them in return. But those with neglect violations tend to be givers attracting takers who never return the attention. People with neglect as their core

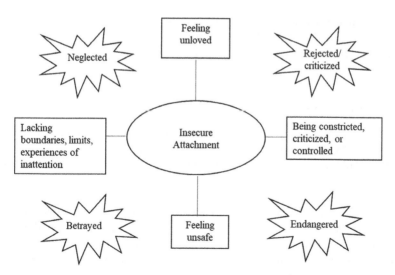

Figure 8.1 Insecure attachment and four types of experiential holograms.

violation may give and give until they feel drained and resentful, and have unconsciously neglected their own needs including time, money, and energy. They are waiting for, but not receiving, the desired love and appreciation. They may also rebuff other's attempts to care for them, by stating they are "fine," "I don't need anything," or, "it is not necessary."

The experiential hologram of emotional neglect is highly prevalent and yet easily missed in psychotherapy. It is not an obvious trauma, or a specific event of trauma but rather a more subtle type of invisible wound, not related to any particular event. It is a form of maltreatment of what did not happen. It may manifest in symptoms of depression, lack of energy, isolation, lack of fulfilling relationships, or symptoms related to lack of self-care. People may also seek therapy for self-destructive behaviors to fill unmet needs such as over-spending, over-eating, engaging in superficial sexual relationships to seek attention, or because they are sabotaging their own goals.

For Amy, she was attentive to others, but quick to neglect her own needs. She sacrificed her own therapy session, thinking that other people's needs are more important than hers. She said as she walked out of the clinic that "her needs are not as important." However, Amy chronically dismisses her own needs, over-cares for others, and feels resentful, drained, and unappreciated. She is lonely and overeats to fill her emotional void.

Amy was the oldest of three sisters and was expected to take care of her siblings while her single mother worked. Amy was always taking care of others while neglecting and ignoring her own needs. At work, she tends to be ignored in staff meetings, but then others ask her to take care of administrative tasks without regard to the buildup of work or the stress that it puts on her. The same dynamic occurs at her church where she gives to exhaustion. In response to her feeling sad and lonely, she tries harder to please and give to others, thereby, keeping her stuck in her holographic cycle.

Rejection trauma

Feeling rejected is deeply painful as it is the trauma of feeling inadequate, not good enough, wrong, and unwanted. It is different from neglect. Where others could simply be preoccupied (and unable to attend to one's needs), with rejection, it is a deliberate act of not wanting or approving of you. This may be typical of a critical parent who focuses on wanting perfection. People with this violation tend to try hard to please others and achieve perfection. They believe that if they are good enough, then maybe they will be accepted and loved. This is of course an illusion as they are already good enough but unconsciously have become their own worst critic and have learned to reject themselves.

Helen was an only child in a military family. Her father, an officer in the Army, was strict at home, and held high expectations for Helen. Helen always felt her father wanted a son and she could never quite meet his approval. She joined the military and served in the Marine Corps to try to impress him. She worked very hard and continued to make rank at a steady pace. However, she was sexually assaulted one night when someone drugged her drink, and her career swiftly ended. She blamed herself and felt like she failed herself, her father, and the military. She put excessive pressure on herself and felt that her only path for redemption was to earn a college degree. She wanted her father to be proud of her and hoped that if she was a straight A student, she would earn rank in his eyes. She was chronically anxious and had put so much pressure on herself that she was not able to focus. She did not meet criteria for ADHD, but rather was suffering from a rejection hologram. She feared not being good enough, tried to be perfect, and was highly self-critical. She feared disappointing others and felt responsible for how her father felt towards her. She wanted his approval/ love and if she didn't get it, it was not only deeply hurtful, but it was her fault. She also negated the achievements that she already had and felt com- pelled to achieve more. However, achievements would likely not get her the emotional outcome that she truly desired.

Betrayal trauma

With betrayal trauma, there is a shattering of a fundamental bond of trust. Those who suffer from this violation may feel they are unable to connect with others or allow themselves to have trusting relationships. Because of a deep sense of loneliness and isolation, they may attempt to trust someone but get into relationships too quickly and suddenly feel betrayed again. People blame themselves and feel they can't trust others, but worst of all, they feel they can't trust themselves or their judgment. Once betrayed, people with this type of trauma may feel angry, distrustful, paranoid, and resentful. They may feel defensive/protective and responsible to detect and catch infidelity before they feel betrayed again. However, they may place unrealistic expectations on others and assume there is betrayal when there may not be.

Samuel presented to therapy angry, defensive, distrustful, and quick to perceive any mishap as a slight against him. When his previous therapist was late, he fired her for disrespecting him. He said he didn't care why she was late; it was her responsibility to be there on time. Samuel said he couldn't remember when his anger and sense of distrust began. He said his sister was manipulative and a liar. As an adult, she spread untruths about him and got other family members to side against him. When his grand- father passed away, she ended up getting all the family money (inheritance) and he got nothing. He felt it was a grave injustice. Now she is trying to be friends with his wife on Facebook. He forbade his wife to talk to her. His wife said she was trying to repair things with the family but Samuel believes his wife betrayed him by sharing pictures with his sister. He accused his wife of lying and trying to sabotage their marriage. He and his wife have been arguing every day until recently she moved out. Samuel feels that everyone is against him, and that he has to protect himself from liars. His fear of distrust was so intense that others felt falsely accused, such as his wife, who didn't trust *him*.

Endangerment trauma

Endangerment trauma occurs in an unhealthy, unpredictable, and abusive environment such as living with someone who abuses alcohol, working under an abusive boss, or being in a violent relationship. Every day is unpredictable—"Will it be safe? Will there be an emotional explosion?" People with this trauma are in a constant state of fear. They also are very alert and attentive to ward off potential danger. Even when they are out of a dangerous situation or relationships, they may continue to expect bad outcomes. People with this hologram never feel safe. In addition, people with this hologram may report that they have all of the other holograms as well. This makes sense because someone who is abusing another person can be both critical and also neglecting, as well as betraying his or her trust. People with this hologram may develop coping responses such as wanting to be in control, or wanting/needing someone else (or something else such as an addiction) to be in control, avoiding relationships or being hyper-sexual having multiple relationships—and at the core of all of these responses is a desire to feel safe and decrease feelings of being unsafe (e.g., safe in relationships, physically, emotionally, and sexually safe).

Also included under this hologram are those who have been a victim of bullying, harassment, and other forms of emotional or psychological abuse. While they may or may not be physically threatened, the mistreatment creates emotional and psychological unsafety. Belittling comments such as someone will never amount to anything, is nihilistic, especially to a vulnerable or budding young person. This type of treatment can make people feel like they are nothing, do not matter, and are unworthy, leaving them feeling empty, insecure/anxious, and/or depressed. A complicating factor is when these comments are delivered in the context of a significant or ongoing relationship (e.g., family, romantic, in school, or work). Positive factors of love, loyalty, and providing livelihood or other factors are mixed-in with the negative comments. People can be rewarded for being "good victims" by taking the abuse and blame (e.g., told they are good, given a present, or a momentary reprieve from the abuse). Pleasing the perpetrator can be deeply intertwined as part of the abuse.

Olivia felt trapped in her family. Not only were her parents, particularly her mother, highly critical and demanding, but her older brother was sexually abusing her. She couldn't stop him or get help from her parents. She thought about betraying her family by asking for outside help but realized it would probably lead to worse outcomes. She feared if she told, her brother would kill her, and it would bring irreparable shame to her family. Her way out was to join the military. Her parents could be proud of her, and she could get herself out of an abusive situation. However, Olivia felt shamed by her family, suffered from severe body distortion (fear of being fat), felt she was never good enough, and had frequent nightmares of sexual abuse (memories of her older brother). She feared going to sleep, feared the night, and feared a home invasion (e.g., someone breaking into her home to rape her). She was not sure if she loved her boyfriend but felt safe when he was there to protect her. Her mother was highly critical of her and put her down. When her mother called, she would adore and praise her brother. It made Olivia feel sick, she wanted to vomit. She literally could not stomach the disgust that she felt with her family. Olivia suffered from an endangerment hologram. In this case, the severe eating disorder needed to be addressed first and she was admitted to a specialized residential treatment program.

Other interpersonal traumas

This discussion would be incomplete without mentioning that there are other interpersonal types of traumas such as being a victim of abuse or maltreatment due to prejudice and discrimination (including but not limited to: racism, sexism, discrimination due to sexual orientation or gender-identity). This type of maltreatment is not only perpetrated by individuals but also by institutions, culture, and systems of authority. It can come from anyone such as a stranger making comments when shopping in a store, to hearing something on the news. It ranges from unconscious bias and stereotypes, micro-aggressive comments, unfair treatment, targeted hate-crimes, to murder, and mass-shootings. It is deeply hurtful, negating, and terrifying. Katz (2005) includes a brief discussion of socio-cultural holograms due to shared trauma and how it could impact large groups of people. Clinicians should assess for (but not assume) client's experiences of discrimination, and the impact it has had on them. These experiences may be part of other interpersonal trauma experiences and may align with any of the four core violations (Table 8.1).

In addition, some trauma is passed down as intergenerational trauma where the origin of the issue occurred with one's parents or grandparents. Identifying the source and releasing "that which is not yours" such as using the catcher's mitt imagery may be helpful (see discussion in Chapter 10). Other forms of maltreatment such as being minimized, not given opportunities, promotions, resources, encouragement, or medical care could

Table 8.1 Types of core violations for interpersonal experiential holograms

Neglected	Rejected	Betrayed	Endangered*
Abandoned	Criticized	Infidelity	Unpredictable danger
Deprived	Judged	Lies/ manipulation	Unsafe
Emotional/physical/ sexual neglect	Compared	Broken promises	Trapped
Ignored	Disdain/ shamed	Deceived/ tricked	Threatened
Dismissed	Invalidated	Unfairly blamed	Dominated
Not loved	Ostracized	Not protected	Controlled
Lack of attention/ care	Excluded/ shunned	Injustice/ unfairness	Emotional/psychological, physical, and sexual abuse
Forgotten	Put down	Taken advantage of	Gas-lighting (abuse + denial or blaming victim)
Overlooked	Refused	Others are disloyal	Name-calling, belittling

* Endangered can include any of the other experiences as well.

potentially fall under any of the other types. More information would be needed to identify if there is a broader pattern.

Components of interpersonal experiential holograms

According to holographic reprocessing, there are six components to an experiential hologram. 1) The *acquired motivation* is the unmet emotional need that motivates actions to engage with others. 2) The *core violation* is the dreaded or feared painful emotional experience. 3) The *personal truth* is the resulting perceptions, feelings, beliefs, operating assumptions, and felt sense about the self, others, and the world. This is the personalized belief of what one's experience means about them. 4) *The compensating coping strategy* is the characteristic response to counteract the perceived negative personal truth. This is a strategy to try to succeed in relationships and attempt to avoid re-experiencing negative affect related to one's hologram. 5) The *avoidance coping strategy* is the behavior used to minimize, avoid, or reduce discomfort. This can be any addiction, emotional eating, or behavior to distract, soothe, or avoid discomfort or painful negative affect related to one's hologram. 6) The *residual emotional state* is the lingering feeling that occurs between cycles of the experiential hologram.

1   Acquired motivation
2   Core violation
3   Personal truth
4   Compensating coping strategies
5   Avoidance coping strategies
6   Residual negative emotions

Acquired motivation

The acquired motivation is an attempt to meet an unmet emotional need. Given basic needs for safety and security including desiring a sense of predictability and control; feeling loved, cared for, attended to; connected with others, or with someone/something beyond oneself; and to feel good about oneself, including self-esteem, and feeling productive and worthy. When emotional needs are unmet, people are left with a desire to meet these needs. The acquired motivation is opposite of one's core violation (the painful pattern of not meeting one's needs).

Core violation

The core violation is the impact of trauma (emotional reaction to an experience) or unmet emotional needs. It is not an event itself such as a robbery or divorce, but rather, what about the event was violating? How did it make the person feel? Four types of interpersonal experiential holograms are offered as core violations: neglected, rejected, betrayed, and endangered. These were developed based on the attachment literature where four factors are associated with secure attachment: feeling loved, safe, having autonomy and self-esteem to explore, and healthy boundaries and limits. When one or more of these factors are insufficient, it could be associated with insecure attachment. Insufficient factors may correspond to interpersonal experiential hologram patterns.

Beliefs about oneself (personal truths)

Epstein (1990) believes we create our own *conception of reality*, or a model of reality, into which we try to make sense of our experiences. This is a desire for parsimony where one's experience and perceptions of the world are aligned and with the goal to meet or sustain basic needs including beliefs that the world is predictable, just, benevolent (Janoff-Bluman, 1992). This is also a striving for control. We want to be able to regulate our environment so our basic emotional and physical needs are satisfied. When we don't know what is going on or have no control such as being in an unpredictable environment, there can be high levels of stress and anxiety, disorientation, confusion, and uncertainty. In times of distress, since children (and adults) are motivated to maintain basic needs of control, connection, and predictability, they will turn towards an explanation that is within their control—themselves. This includes thoughts of what they could have done or should have done, who they are, how they contributed or caused outcomes, or self-blame for ongoing experiences.

Compensating coping strategies

Compensating strategies are behaviors to try to counteract one's experiential hologram and it is typically the opposite of one's beliefs about the self. If someone believes they are not good enough, then they may compensate by trying to be perfect. While it is a laudable attempt to undo the hologram, it is ineffective. It is the opposite side of the same coin, but still part of the coin. Even with outstanding compensation behaviors, the belief is still intact, and therefore, so is the experiential hologram. It is not until the personalized beliefs are called into question, that the hologram will be lifted.

Avoidance coping strategies

Avoidance coping strategies are present with all types of holograms and can range from non-problematic distracting or calming behaviors to very problematic behaviors that need treatment or immediate intervention. On the healthy or non-destructive end of the continuum, the word avoidance may be inaccurate and too narrow, as it is adaptive to release, disengage, or diffuse from negative affective states. These strategies may help moderate and manage stress. Examples include watching a television show or movie, playing an occasional video game, having a single bowl of ice-cream or single drink of alcohol, taking an occasional nap, going out to a club or casino on occasion for entertainment, engaging in a hobby, exercising, talking to a friend, deep breathing, going for a hike, going shopping, cooking, cleaning, going for a drive, or meditating.

Moderate problematic behaviors may have initially served to manage stress but have become problematic and depending on severity would need treatment. This includes on the continuum of more than occasional to excessive use: of television or video games to the exclusion of other activities, eating resulting in unwanted weight gain or eating disorders, use of alcohol, drugs, nicotine, caffeine, excessive sleep, gambling, use of pornography, spending money, exercise, or other behaviors used to the exclusion of other activities, causing disruption in relationship, time, health, or finances and not stopping even when the behavior is causing problems.

This can also include emotionally shutting down, isolating from others, withdrawing from relationships, and thoughts of suicide. For some, depression can be a response to feeling so overwhelmed and hopeless that they cannot deal with life stressors. Other strategies could be getting into fights, engaging in superficial sexual relationships, risk taking, impulsive acts, and running away from situations (e.g., quitting, relocating, or abruptly ending relationships).

Severe problematic behaviors include actions or plans that endangers oneself or others. It could include any of the strategies mentioned above but to a severe level causing significant disruption such as legal actions, significant damage, and possibly irreparable damage to self and/or other.

Because everyone has the need for stress management, affect management, and/or avoidance of negative affective states, emotion regulation skills are offered as part of holographic reprocessing treatment. The extent of attention needed for affect management can be tailored to client needs.

An efficient way to understand the complex components of an experiential hologram is through the template of a pot on the stove—heating up, steaming, and possibly boiling over is a way of illustrating how holograms activate and cycle. There are six elements: Knobs to turn on the heat, the burner that heats up the stove, the pot itself sitting on the burner, the

Table 8.2 Overview of four types of interpersonal experiential holograms

	Neglected	Rejected	Betrayed	Endangered
Private beliefs about myself	I'm unwanted, not important, insignificant, alone. My needs don't matter	I'm not good enough. Worries of being judged, inadequate, or failing	I'm gullible, easily taken advantage of. People lie, are untrustworthy	I'm not safe, I'm nothing, I'm bad, out of control, others are dangerous
Compensating strategies	Be wanted: being helpful, funny, attentive to others, sexy, overcaring of others	Be perfect: critical of self and others, high expectations, seek perfection	Be wary: not trusting others, being suspicious of others	Be safe: being submissive, or in control, avoiding conflict, trying to please/agree/ help others to avoid upset
Chronic residual emotions	Depression: tired, drained, lonely	Anxiety: worried, fear of failure	Anger: resentful, paranoid	Fear: hypervigilant, frantic, panic, overwhelmed
Motivation	To feel cared for, appreciated, attended to	To feel accepted, included, acknowledged	To feel secure, have loyalty, trust	To feel safe and secure, free from danger

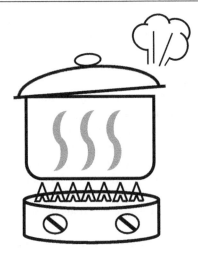

Figure 8.2 The pot on a stove is a template to map the six components on an experiential hologram.

contents boiling inside the pot, a lid, and steam coming out of the lid. The pot on the stove is a template with each part of the image corresponding to a specific element of the hologram. The components of the hologram can be mapped via an interactive discussion with clients to identify patterns using the template of a pot on the stove.

The **knobs on the stove** correspond to needs that were not met during one's life that may initiate or motivate the holographic cycle. This is the acquired motivation which is the desire to relieve negative feelings brought on by the hologram. The motivation is typically to engage in a positive relationship. They are seeking to fulfill basic needs such as security, relatedness, and self-esteem. In other words, people want to feel safe, loved, and good about themselves.

The **hot burner** corresponds to the **core violation** or emotional pain; it is the essence of what is feared or dreaded, such as being neglected, rejected, betrayed, or endangered, yet may be replicated repeatedly.

The **contents of the pot** correspond to the thoughts and feelings about the self, others, and the world. These beliefs are the personalized truths or what one comes to believe about oneself. They are acquired from past experiences, although they do not have to be true as one moves into the future. Examples are "I'm not good enough," "I don't matter," "I'm insignificant," "I'm stupid," "I'm unworthy," "the world is not safe," "I can't trust anyone," and "all people want to harm me."

The **lid on the pot** is an attempt to contain the boiling contents, and corresponds to ways of coping. These include avoidance strategies and compensating strategies. The compensating coping strategy is the typical way a person counteracts or compensates for the negative self-perceptions and feelings produced by the personal truths. However, as long as the personal truth is believed to be true, the compensating strategies are never convincing enough and never bring enough comfort to the painful underlying feelings. As the term suggests, it is a compensating strategy and does not heal or fix the personal truth. In fact, it is usually a rigid and ineffective strategy that inadvertently facilitates the replication of the dreaded violation. People's compensating strategies are usually a positive quality (such as being helpful, funny, in control, attending to details, advocating for oneself, etc.) but it is rigid behavior where the person feels compelled to do these things or otherwise feels guilty, anxious, out of control, or unsafe.

The **steam** that escapes from the pot corresponds to the **residual negative emotions** that linger between cycles of the hologram. This is usually a negative feeling that may instigate strategies to relieve the discomfort caused by this state. Some typical residual emotional states are feelings such as being lonely, needy, insecure, or anxious. For example, people may feel resentment after they give and give in a relationship that ends up being neglectful.

Example of a "pot on the stove" for a neglect hologram

- Burner *core violation:* Neglected, abandoned, dismissed, ignored
- Boiling contents *beliefs (Personal truth):* I'm not important, my needs don't matter
- Lid *compensating strategy:* Please others, attend to their needs to earn love
- Lid *avoidance strategy:* Depression, neglect of one's own needs, isolation from others
- Steam *residual negative emotions:* Lonely, drained, tired, depressed
- Knobs *acquired motivation:* Secure love, attention, appreciation

Example of a "pot on the stove" for a rejection hologram

- Burner *core violation:* Rejected, disapproved, judged
- Boiling contents *beliefs (Personal truth):* I'm not good enough, feeling inadequate
- Lid *compensating strategy:* Perfectionism, criticize, judge, or reject self and others
- Lid *avoidance strategy:* Try harder, or avoid activities and social events
- Steam *residual negative emotions:* Anxious, worried
- Knobs *acquired motivation:* Acceptance

Example of a "pot on the stove" for a betrayal hologram

- Burner *core violation:* Betrayed, lied to, broken trust
- Boiling contents *beliefs (personal truth):* I'm stupid/gullible, others are not trustworthy

- Lid *compensating strategy:* Be wary, don't trust/tend to be very loyal and trusting
- Lid *avoidance strategy:* Defensive towards others, distrustful
- Steam *Residual negative emotions:* resentment, bitter, angry
- Knobs *acquired motivation:* Seek loyal relationships

Example of a "pot on the stove" for an endangerment hologram

- Burner *core violation:* Endangered, trapped, oppressed, threatened
- Boiling contents *beliefs (personal truth):* I'm unsafe, life is out of control/chaotic
- Lid *compensating strategy:* Be in control/take charge or be submissive/disappear
- Lid *avoidance strategy:* Avoid conflict or upset, be submissive, over-caring
- Steam *residual negative emotions:* Anxious, fearful, hypervigilant, on-edge
- Knobs *acquired motivation:* Security, predictability, and control

Chapter summary

This chapter explained the four main clusters of interpersonal experiential holograms: neglect, rejection/criticism, betrayal, and endangerment. The six components of the holograms were presented using the template of a pot on the stove.

Chapter 9

Other trauma-based experiential holograms

This chapter outlines experiential holograms incurred from experiences of moral injury, life-threatening trauma or being a victim of a crime, and complicated grief. These experiences can render a person stuck, as if frozen in time, with a gnawing unresolved hologram unable to process or resolve the past.

Case example: The night we both died

Henry was an African-American male with PTSD and depression, who served in the military. He was stationed on an aircraft carrier. He said he usually keeps things to himself, and others understand (e.g., his wife, family, and friends) that he is irritable and likes to be alone. He has nightmares, poor sleep, vivid intrusive thoughts about the military, and depression. His primary care providers referred him for mental health assessment and he was referred to sleep medicine to be evaluated for sleep apnea.

Henry looked depressed. He had difficulty smiling (constricted affect), dysphoric mood, pessimistic thinking, and a slow heaviness about him. His wife says he is overly sensitive and moody. He has difficulty concentrating. He was not on any medications for mood or sleep. He said as he gets older, his memory is so vivid. He said ever since his service he's been angry and upset. His friends at his church told him it was never too late to get help, so he agreed to meet with a counselor, although he was pessimistic. We discussed memory and his preoccupation with the past and how he is pulled into the past versus being fully present (e.g., driving while looking in the rearview mirror metaphor). We discussed that his rearview mirror was nightmares and intrusive thoughts from the military.

The main trauma event for him occurred one day when he was walking on the deck of an aircraft carrier. It was raining and windy. He had to be in a certain place on the flight deck to launch a plane. He was talking with an acquaintance who was walking ahead of him. Henry said as they were

DOI: 10.4324/9781003223429-11

talking, the acquaintance casually moved to the left and didn't see there was a spinning propeller. Henry witnessed him walk into the spinning propeller. The vision haunts him, and he can't put it out of his mind. He wakes up screaming in his sleep. He has a lot of anxiety about planes, particularly propeller planes.

We discussed that he has complicated traumatic grief. He said he thinks about the conditions that lead up to the event: wearing heavy duty ear muffs, in the rain with the wind, walking around the propeller planes that were not protected. The propellers were going at a speed making them invisible. And his friend's guard was down just for a second... he feels haunted thinking if only he could have saved him. For his treatment plan, we agreed on addressing three things: his sleep including night-mares (and possible treatments depending on the results from his sleep test), depression (including a medication consultation for his depression), and complicated grief.

We started with addressing his sleep habits and recurrent nightmares. After discussing the content of his nightmare, he agreed to engage in ima-gery rescripting. He came up with a positive image to replace his nightmare. In subsequent sessions, he reported reduced frequency of nightmares, and then none.

Given his initial success, he was open to using a similar procedure to rescript and reprocess images of the past. He had intrusive memories where the past was intruding on the present instead of floating into the past where it belongs. We discussed his spiritual beliefs about what hap-pens after death. He said he was a strong Christian and believes souls go to heaven. He said he prays for the soul of his acquaintance, that his soul is resting in peace.

We discussed if there was anything he wanted to communicate to him. He said he was sorry his life ended that day. He said that man was a poor soul who lost his life, but we discussed that Henry also lost a part of his life that day, by being stuck with him for all these years. What happened to his friend, in a way also happened to him. By visualizing his friend being free, visualizing his soul going up to heaven like a dove flying into the sky, also frees him. They were both stuck, but now they can both be free. He could see that it was an accident, not his fault, although he wished it had not happened. We discussed being careful of his negative thinking and regrets as this brings him down and he can't do anything about the past. He cannot change it. But rather, he can work on allowing the past to be in the past, seeing his friend's soul lifting up and remembering that he is free. This shifts the recall from being in it (as if re-experiencing the horror) to rising above it, seeing it from a new perspective where his friend's soul is peaceful and free. In turn, allowing the client's soul to also be peaceful and free.

After this reprocessing, we discussed focusing on the present and his future. We discussed what can he do now that would be meaningful. He said what is meaningful is to volunteer to help other veterans. He said he thinks it will make him feel good to help other veterans. In addition, it will help him socialize more. He acknowledged that he does feel better when he is engaged in activities.

Henry worked on his imagery, got treatment for sleep apnea, started on medication for mood, and increased his activity level. His depression improved, noted no nightmares for the past couple of sessions, and he is focused on being present and future-oriented in a meaningful way. And when he thinks about that event, he shifts his attention to seeing his friend's soul at peace and free.

Additional types of experiential holograms

Other experiential holograms acquired from trauma or intense emotional experiences may include unresolved or lingering thoughts and beliefs particularly around blame secondary to moral injury, experiences of trauma (including sexual trauma), and complicated grief or losses. Like interpersonal experiential holograms, they may have at their core, personalized beliefs such as, "It's my fault." These beliefs may be altered by considering context. The hologram may also be addressed through imagery reprocessing tailored to the needs of the client.

Trauma is broadly defined in holographic reprocessing, and may include witnessing or experiencing life-threatening events, or potential life-threatening events including experiencing painful or invasive medical issues, but could also include non-life-threatening emotionally significant events such as harassment, emotional abuse, costly or frustrating legal battles, or abrupt or significant losses. It is a significant event that has left a holographic imprint and source of intrusive thoughts, personalized beliefs, and emotional symptoms.

Moral-injury-based experiential holograms

Moral injury occurs in response to perpetrating, failing to prevent, or witnessing actions that go against one's individual values and/or moral beliefs (Litz et al., 2009). There is an unresolved incongruity, or dissonance between one's actions and one's morals, with a lingering feeling of regret, self-blame, disgust, and/or grief. Given the motivation to make sense of discrepancies, people may conclude that they are unworthy, bad, guilty, and not only deserve to be punished, but deserve to never be forgiven. Thus, they will likely reject suggestions of self-forgiveness and may suffer from prolonged self-deprecation, depression, or desire for self-harm. Even efforts to seek a spiritual resolution may be rebuffed.

Examples are committing acts of violence against others including killing in war, witnessing others violating ethical behavior, and either contributing to or not stopping it, having to function under unethical or immoral leadership, or committing acts that knowingly violate one's moral beliefs and values. For example, Abe is a client who cheated on this wife and lives with unremitting guilt and shame. In these trauma holograms, the personalization that they are guilty is objectively true, it is not a distortion. But what is a distortion is being stuck to the point of dysfunction and thwarting any efforts of healing or growth. Forgiveness is a slippery concept and may be seen as negating or simply washing away the guilt, when guilt feels appropriate and consistent with one's values. The guilt feels right because the behavior was wrong.

Utilizing holographic reprocessing principles, these cases may be helped by offering a contextual perspective. Context can help lift someone out of their own limited point of view. It may open up a new perception (e.g., such as considering the context) or help to consider what others may need, feel, or want. For Abe, the question is, what does his wife and his family need from him now? How can he contribute to healing, repairing, and helping his family? He values his family and would like to move towards his value of wanting to be a good father/husband. He has already went to years of therapy, and has made many apologies. But his depression and constant guilt only pulls attention away from his family, and keeps the focus on him. This only perpetuates his self-centeredness. Instead, the focus shifts from, "I am a terrible person," to how can I care for or support the needs of someone else.

> Broadening perspective creates room to entertain new ways to make sense of moral injury experiences. This may be coupled with letter writing, imagery reprocessing, considering reparative actions, and focusing on the future.

Not everyone will be open to shifting or forgiving oneself, so this is a delicate conversation of both acknowledging the trauma and/or wrong doing and offering a palatable way to move forward. For example, a veteran who served in a war, told his team to kill civilians who were planting explosives on the roads to harm Americans. He not only felt justified but highly motivated to "get them." However, once they were killed, he was mortified. He said he didn't want therapy and he would never, ever, forgive himself. For him, his guilt was his punishment and it was his burden to bear. He did not want to see it any other way.

Finally, moral injury could be in part due to a limited perspective, as in the opening case examples for Chapters 3 and 10. In both of these examples, once the clients considered context, they realized what happened was not their fault. After treatment, they no longer had a moral injury, and were able to grieve losses to resolve their pasts.

These types of trauma issues are complex with multiple perspectives. The Kleenex tissue box metaphor can be helpful to see different aspects of the same situation. What were the motives, agenda, context for each person at the time of the event? When reconsidering the event, now in a different time and context, what might have made sense under certain conditions, may not make sense once out of those conditions. We are complex human beings and we are meant to learn, grow, and evolve. While it may be appropriate to regret some actions, it is also appropriate to grieve, acknowledge, come to terms with what is and was, and make concerted reparative actions. Lamenting about the past does not fix or change it. It is occupying time that could be used more productively.

Trauma from being a victim of a crime, or other threatening event

When people experience an unwanted life event or trauma, they will inevitably review the event and wonder why this terrible thing happened to them and what could they have done differently to prevent it. They may engage in if-only thinking (e.g., if only I did this instead of that...). Even when the event is clearly due to the actions of an assailant such as being robbed, or assaulted (even if they were drugged and unconscious), they may still wonder what they could have, or should have done differently and may therefore, conclude, "This is my fault." They may regret events that occurred before or leading up to the trauma and blame themselves for not knowing, not acting, not screaming, fighting, reporting, turning right or left, or somehow not preventing it. People can be stuck with this type of self-blame and thwart efforts to heal because deep inside they still blame themselves.

Examples are victims of sexual assault, victims of crime, victims of a partner's infidelity ("it's my fault they cheated on/left me"), and/or self-blame for poor outcomes with one's children ("it's my fault my child turned out to be a drug addict"). This type of self-blame is accurately related to regret and grief for poor outcomes, but it is inaccurately related to one's culpability. This type of self-blame fails to consider context.

As discussed in chapter 3, it takes a thief for a theft to occur. Regardless of what the wallet is doing, even if it's full of money, or drunk on a table, there will not be a theft without a thief. A thief knowingly plans and executes a theft, and then tries to get away with it. The theft occurs because of the thief, not the wallet. In fact, it is impossible for the wallet to thieve itself. Someone may argue that the wallet shouldn't have been there, or the wallet should have fought back. The wallet wouldn't have to worry about where it was, or fighting at all, if it wasn't being attacked. The discussion is about putting blame where blame is due. And letting people be responsible for their own actions. The person may have regretted putting their wallet down, but that is not the cause of the theft. If a thief really wants a wallet, they can find a way to get it. It is impossible to try to predict or control other people's behavior. What a thief chooses to do is not the wallet's fault. Similarly, if someone chooses to engage in infidelity, that is their choice and their behavior. Other people's choices are theirs. This addresses the issue of responsibility and blame. Imagery may include reprocessing where one's current-age self visits the younger self to let them know it wasn't their fault. Once addressed, there may be other issues such as grief and acknowledging losses.

Another type of trauma-based experiential hologram can form from a dangerous or life-threatening experience. This includes recovery from a car or other accident, medical trauma incurred from having to go through invasive procedures or a life-threatening diagnosis, being mugged or threatened, or any near-miss dangerous or threatening event. This is addressed through the hindsight advantage strategy (Katz, 2005), where the current-age self knows the outcome and can reassure the younger self that they are going to be okay. The younger self may be terrified but the current-age self can whisper in their ear, "You're going to be okay." This helps the younger self relax and release the pent-up traumatic fear.

This shifts the memory from the field vantage point as if reliving the experience of life-threatening danger to the observer vantage point. Using the hindsight advantage, one can see self in context, and the bigger story. Clients can create their own imagery to let their younger self know it's going to be okay (e.g., imagine leaving the situation, reassuring one's younger self, or leaving a gift or symbol for the younger self from the current self to remind them they will be okay). This changes the hologram.

Complicated grief-based experiential holograms

Complicated grief is grief that does not resolve naturally. Acknowledging that losses, including deaths, require time for assimilation, the grieving process may include a period of disorientation and disbelief before coming to acceptance and readjusting to a new reality (Shear et al., 2007). This process may continue over several years, changing and unfolding as people process through their thoughts and feelings. However, complicated grief doesn't seem to resolve but rather seems to be stuck. People may have ongoing repetitive intrusive thoughts, thoughts of self-blame, regrets, and if-only thinking which maintains and impedes grief resolution. They may toggle between guilt, longing, sadness, and feeling that they can't live their life or be happy because of what happened to them or someone else.

A further complication is disenfranchised grief which is not openly acknowledged or supported by others or society. A common example is after the loss of a pet, or a miscarriage, someone may say, "Oh well, have another," which negates and minimizes one's hurt and loss. But there are many experiences that have layers of associated losses with ongoing repercussions, some aspects acknowledged and other layers are left to be quietly mourned in isolation. With these experiences there can be a deep, gut-wrenching sense of helplessness, hurt, longing, anger, loneliness among other reactions and an unrelenting wish or desire to change, control, or stop the event. It is heavy, depressing, and may lead to overwhelming persistent grief. Some may have thoughts of suicide themselves to escape the pain or turn towards pain-relieving substance use. It is compounded when others don't seem to understand, or want the person to get over it, and seem to minimize the impact of the experience.

One client had been grieving the loss of his younger sister for several years. He came to therapy worried about an upcoming family gathering and didn't think he could handle being around his family. His sister was assaulted as a teenager and ran away from home. She never came back but would text their mother on occasion to let them know she was okay. One day they got a call that she had died in an accident. The client blamed himself for not helping or saving his sister and has been stuck in grief ever since.

We worked on seeing things from the other person's point of view. In the case above, we discussed that his sister lived on her own terms. She refused to be confined. We acknowledged her courage. The meta-reframe was that his sister chose freedom, embraced her power, and lived on her own terms which was quite remarkable for someone so young. The client said he hadn't thought of that, but it fits. It made him feel better about his sister's choice. For the imagery reprocessing, the client was asked if he had a communication he wanted to deliver to his sister. In grief imagery, we work on letting people be free, seeing their souls releasing, and creating imagery that is culturally consistent with the beliefs of the client. In the case above, the client imagined being with his sister, in spirit form. She put her hand on the client's shoulder and said, "It's okay." The client felt his sister was telling him that she's okay, and it's okay for him to move forward and live his life. The client said it really helped him and he looked forward to spending time with his family. We also discussed ways for the client to focus on living his life and finding ways to honor his sister moving forward.

Complicated grief is about completing communications, allowing people to be on their own journey, visualizing lost one's souls being free, releasing guilt, blame, shame, and ultimately coming to terms with what is. It is important to note, that sometimes there are no words to make a horrible, tragic, or senseless event okay. It is not okay. Sometimes what is needed is someone to share a painful experience, bear witness, validate, provide empathy, and offer comfort. During imagery reprocessing, the client or client with the therapist can stand by the traumatized self, to say, "I am with you, you are not alone."

Table 9.1 Experiential holograms: Moral injury, victim of trauma, and complicated grief

	Moral injury (inflicted on others, witnessed, or participated in trauma)	Victim of crime or trauma (incl. assault, abuse, harassment, infidelity)	Complicated grief
Emotional reactions	Appropriate guilt (anger, disgust, regret) for what I did do (contributed to it, participated, witnessed, didn't stop it, or even initiated it)	Inappropriate guilt, blaming self for what others did/as if it could have been prevented (if-only thinking)	Distorted guilt for what could have or should have happened, if-only thinking, unresolved longing, mourning, regret
Perceptions about blame	Resistant to self-forgiveness because guilt is congruous with their morals and values	Consider putting blame where blame is due, allowing others to be responsible for their own actions	Consider event from the other person's perspective, allowing them to be on their own journey, making their own choices
Context for blame/ and understanding	Instead focus on seeing context, perhaps self-forgiveness, finding meaning/purpose, and identifying reparations to others, reinventing oneself/ commit to values, may need to address grief	Usually open to self-forgiveness once they put blame where blame is due. Also, may need to address anger, resentments, and grief	Imagine expressing whatever the client wants to express to the deceased, seeing context, letting each person have their life journey whatever it may be. Find things to appreciate
Type of imagery	Imagery for releasing guilt, grief, communicating with younger self, or deceased if appropriate. Focus on doing something productive, healing, and reparative	Imagery for self-compassion, releasing self-blame, visiting younger self, providing comfort, reassurance, not their fault, they are going to be okay	Imagery of communicating with younger self (not their fault) or deceased if appropriate. Seeing others as free. Focus on releasing, reparative efforts, and comforting imagery

Summary of trauma-based experiential holograms

The trauma-based experiential holograms mentioned above have in common a persistence as if the person is frozen in time, unable to process or resolve the past experience. It may reoccur as intrusive thoughts, nightmares, trauma-related emotional triggers (as if re-experiencing a familiar feeling), or as if it is always playing in the background, just below the surface of awareness. Something may happen that brings the memory forward, or is similar enough to initiate a cascade of emotions and physical reactions. These holograms are visual and sensory (not encoded as language) and can have a pervasive impact on one's well-being. People feel stuck. For those who find that recalling and reliving the events as if it were happening to them does not help (but rather reinforces and re-traumatizes them), then considering the observer vantage point may offer room to find a new way out. This facilitates understanding context and considering other people's agendas and other perspectives. This lays the foundation for imagery reprocessing.

In this chapter's opening case example, Henry was stuck reliving the horrific image of his friend walking into the propeller. Henry felt helpless and guilty because he couldn't help him. But he shifted by viewing the event from a different perspective where he focused on his soul being free. In the original image his friend was not okay, but in the second image, his friend's soul was okay. This gave him a way out from being stuck.

Chapter summary

This chapter presents details about other types of experiential holograms that are common responses to trauma experiences such as moral injury, being a victim of a crime, experience of a life-threatening event, and complicated grief. Each of these holograms has unique associated responses regarding blame, guilt, and what they need for healing.

Chapter 10

Considering context

This chapter presents the rationale and several strategies and metaphors to shift perception, meaning, and understanding of one's past. Experiential holograms are formed in a context. Utilizing the observer vantage point, the context of circumstance, one's age, and other's agendas are revealed to see a broader more comprehensive picture.

Case example: A small piece in a large machine

Marcus was a male veteran referred by his primary care provider for major depression. However, when he came to the appointment, he said it would be "useless." He said he has been in therapy many times and has tried numerous medications. Thinking this would be a brief assessment, I asked him a simple question, when did the depression start? He gave me a specific date. At that point, I knew what the problem was. Everyone was treating depression, but depression doesn't start on a specific date. Trauma does. He likely had unresolved trauma that nobody had addressed. Something happened on that day, and I hypothesized to him, that what happened on that date is what needed to be addressed.

I asked, "What happened?" He said that's the date when he opened the file. He said he shouldn't have ever opened that file. "What was in the file?" I asked. "Pictures," he replied. They were pictures of people who died from a bombing released from a vehicle that he fixed. Marcus blamed himself for this awful tragedy because he was the one who fixed the vehicle. He believed that if he hadn't fixed it, then the bombing would not have occurred. He said they didn't tell him what they were going to use it for when they asked him to fix it. When he saw the pictures, a part of him shut down from a tremendous sense of guilt. No antidepressant was going to help him after that.

I told him that I thought he was having a trauma response. I proposed that we could address this in 4–6 sessions. I explained my approach and he said it sounded, "intriguing." He was interested in engaging in the process. We discussed more details about the incident. He had specialized mechanic

DOI: 10.4324/9781003223429-12

skills and nobody else in his unit could have fixed the vehicle. In his mind, he was the one who enabled this tragedy to happen. It was his actions which led to this outcome.

We discussed context. There were many decisions and many meetings that occurred before he was asked to fix the vehicle. We can only speculate on the details, but what we do know is that someone planned this attack, and several people made decisions to carry it out. Fixing vehicles was the veteran's job. He did his job and did it well. He had orders to do his job. But this was in a context of many people who participated, on both sides.

The veteran said he understood. He was only a small piece in a large machine. It was not his fault any more than anyone else in the entire machine. We also discussed seeing his younger self who was motivated to do a good job. We also don't know how many lives were potentially saved by the mission. Finally, we discussed grieving the loss of innocent life. We did an imagery of seeing their souls being free.

He said for over ten years he had thought about this incident nearly daily. In a follow-up session, he said he stopped thinking about it. Two months later, he said, "You have done more for me than anyone else has ever done." His guilt and intrusive thoughts had resolved. The part of him that was frozen in time had thawed. Now he thinks about present issues and planning for the future. His pre- to post-treatment test scores decreased considerably from severe to minimal on ratings of depression, and PTSD, and from moderate to mild on his ratings of anxiety.

Field vs observer vantage point when recalling memories

This case example illustrated that despite numerous medications and treatments, this veteran's depression was not resolving, and likely would not, until his perception about what happened changed. He blamed himself for what happened as if it was his actions that lead to the horrific outcome. He had a moral injury and was horrified by what he did. It violated his conscience. He regretted participating in an act that went against his own moral values and he said he regretted participating in the military.

It is accurate that he did participate in a critical part of carrying out this mission. But what was not accurate was his narrow perspective of the event. His personalization lacked context. He recalled the memory as if he was in it, recalling details as if they were happening, and seeing events as if through his eyes at the time of his experience. This is the field vantage point. Like a field mouse in the grass, all the mouse can see are the blades of grass in front of him. However, to gain perspective, it is necessary to widen the lens, see a bigger picture, and lift out of the experience. From the view of an objective observer, a bigger picture is revealed. This is the observer vantage point, like an eagle flying above, the eagle can see the mouse and the context of the entire field. But the mouse cannot. Like a field mouse, this veteran could only see what he had done and the results that ensued. His perception lacked the context that only an eagle can see.

McIsaac and Eich (2002, 2004) studies demonstrated differences in recall from the field and observer vantage points. In their 2002 study, after manipulating objects, students were asked to recall their experience from one of the two vantage points. Those recalling from the field vantage point remarked about their affective reactions, physical sensations, and emotional states (e.g., how they felt at the time as if reliving the experience). In contrast, those who recalled their experience from the observer vantage point remarked on their personal appearance, actions they made, and spatial relations among objects in the room (e.g., as if watching themselves in the context of the room). Similarly, in their second study, when patients with PTSD recalled memories from the field vantage point, their associated emotional responses were more negative and more intense (more anxiety provoking) than when the memories were recalled from the observer vantage point (McIsaac & Eich, 2004).

These findings have been replicated in several related studies. Akhtar et al., (2017) found that field vantage point memories were more vivid, emotionally intense and more personally important than observer memories. In their study, they asked participants to switch their vantage point. When memories originally recalled as observer memories were then recalled from the field perspective, there was no change, but when memories originally recalled as field memories were then recalled from the observer perspective there was marked reduction in vivid details. Wisco et al. (2015) also found that when participants adopted an observer vantage point to recall memories, they had low physiological reactivity compared to those in the field/immersed condition who had increased heart rate and skin conductance responses. Mooren et al. (2019) tested vantage point recall in a laboratory setting inducing recall of images of a traumatic car accident. Recall from the field perspective resulted in higher negative mood, anxiety, and more intrusions compared to those in the observer condition and control condition.

In contrast, Kenny et al. (2009) in a large prospective study, found that more severe PTSD symptoms were related to recalling trauma from an observer vantage point at an initial time period and at 12 months later. They contend that adopting an observer perspective directly after the traumatic event (i.e., during memory consolidation) might be effective in dampening initial emotional arousal and preventing intrusion development, but when the memory is already consolidated, adopting an observer perspective might function as an avoidance strategy that eventually maintains PTSD symptoms. In contrast, Akhtar et al. (2017) found that recent memories tended to be recalled from the field vantage point, while consolidated remote memories of childhood were predominately recalled from the observer perspective, and these were associated with low levels of distress.

For the participants in the Kenny et al. (2009) study, high levels of avoidance may be addressed by recalling details of trauma from the field vantage point to help process feared content for desensitization. This is consistent with prolonged exposure (PE) therapy. In the case example, Marcus was diagnosed with depression but also met criteria for PTSD. He had indirect exposure to aversive details of the trauma incurred in the course of his professional duties and had excessive self-blame. While exposure therapy may be helpful for those with high avoidance, it would not be helpful for Marcus. Avoidance was not what was maintaining his symptoms, nor would further recall from a field vantage point help him, either. In fact, he said he thought about his experience daily for ten years. He was stuck in his recall from the field vantage point. For him, the observer vantage point facilitated a new perspective. This helped him consider factors outside of himself.

Holographic reprocessing is not limited to PTSD events (exposure to death, threatened death, actual or threatened serious injury, or actual or threatened sexual violence). From the holographic reprocessing perspective, there are a range of traumatic or intense experiences that may or may not meet PTSD criteria leading to a variety of symptoms. The events addressed in holographic reprocessing have in common a sense of being stuck due to a limited perception, personalization, or self-blame. While PE may address anxiety and trauma symptoms maintained by avoidance, once this is addressed, clients may still benefit from considering context, especially if they have unresolved issues of self-blame, resentment, and/or grief:

An anxiety-based trauma associated with avoidance, emotional dysregulation, and lack of trauma integration, could be more appropriate for a field-based recall using exposure.

An experiential hologram associated with a personalized perception which maintains symptoms, could be more appropriate for an observer-based recall to consider context.

In summary, the observer vantage point facilitates:

• Emotional distance from the event
• Seeing a broader context
• Holistic reappraisal of event, meaning, and personal truths (e.g., "it's my fault.")

Strategies for reappraisal

Utilizing the observer vantage point, several strategies can be used to facilitate reappraisals such as: 1) multiple points of view (including age comparison), 2) reframes and meta-reframes, and 3) strategies for disengaging from the trauma. These reappraisals are not about shifting specific automatic thoughts such as addressing problematic thinking in CPT, but rather to overall perceptions and meanings.

Multiple points of view

Multiple points of view allow for a complex understanding of an event without refuting someone's experience. It suggests that the client's perception is true and accurate for the client, but there may be more to the picture. A metaphor is offered using a tissue box (e.g., Kleenex) where the client may be able to see one side (let's say it is blue), and may not be aware of the color of the opposite side of the box (e.g., that is red). From one perspective, the client can only see one side of the box. However, once the other sides are revealed, the client can see there is a blue and red side, and maybe a yellow and purple side too. This is particularly helpful in couple therapy, as both participants have an accurate perception given their perspective of the box. One is not right while the other is wrong, but rather there are multiple rights, or multiple truths. These multiple perspectives may be both simultaneously contradictory and accurate.

Multiple points of view allow others to consider the same story from other people's perspective. What might they be responding to from their own past? One of the philosophies of holographic reprocessing is that everyone makes sense from their own perspective. Most people believe they are right, their thoughts make sense, and their choices feel right to them based on their own perceptions, thoughts, and feelings. The strategy of multiple points of view is not about agreeing with the other perspectives, but rather understanding that they exist.

One of the techniques with multiple points of view is to have clients write a trauma story or event from the perspective of everyone who was involved. What were their motives, agendas, perspectives? This helps people see that those who were purposefully plotting to harm had their own agenda. This allows perpetrators of abuse to be responsible for their own actions. From an expanded view, it is easier to more accurately assign blame where it is due. It helps open a discussion of blame and responsibility.

Age comparison

Another strategy discussed in Katz (2005) is age comparison. In this technique, people consider the ages of themselves and others at the time of their trauma. This allows the current-age self to gain a new perspective on the younger aged self as well as everyone else involved. To gain perspective on perpetrators, a client is asked how old the perpetrator was in the scene and this age is compared to the client's current age. The example in Katz (2005) was a client named Leslie whose parents divorced when she was three. She remembers hearing that her father didn't want her. She was devastated by this and subsequently had a history of failed relationships with men who left her. When asked about the ages of her parents, she said her mother had her when she was only 19 years old, and her father was 20 years old. Apparently, her father, who was not ready to be married nor a father, felt trapped when her mother got pregnant. Now that Leslie is 30 years old, she was able to have a new understanding about her father's feelings as a 20-year-old. Age comparison helps clients to see their parents from the perspective of a peer rather than as authority figures. She could release her anger towards her father and see his limitations– she said, "Now, I feel compassion for him." She could also have compassion for her younger self who always tried so hard, and felt unlovable.

To broaden the clients' view of their younger self, they are asked to identify the age they were at the time of the trauma. Then, they are asked to find someone who is that age to remind them of what it was like to be that age. Most are surprised to see how innocent others are at their younger age. Another example from Katz (2005) is a 53-year-old client who worked the night shift on a burn unit. Unfortunately, many died on her shift. She blamed herself for not saving more lives. However, when she considered her age at the time of being 19 years old, fresh out of a two-year nursing school, she at 53, could have more compassion for her young self. The perspective achieved with age comparison can only be garnered retrospectively.

Perspective can only be achieved retrospectively.

Hindsight advantage

This strategy is reviewing a past event with the knowledge of how it is going to turn out. When someone is in the moment of a life-threatening event, they do not know what will happen and may be flooded with fear. Recalling the event from the field vantage point with knowledge about how threatening the situation really was, only intensifies the associated fear. However, reprocessing the experience with hindsight advantage means they know the outcome, they know they are going to survive and be okay. For example, Nick was in a motorcycle accident and since then has had intrusive images of seeing his front wheel hit a piece of concrete on the road. He thinks about if he had fallen slightly to the left, the bike would have crushed him. When he recalls the event, he thinks about how he could have died.

Instead, with the hindsight advantage strategy, he imagined his current-age self at the scene telling his younger self he is going to be fine. He said, "You're going to walk away from this." He told his therapist, "I must have had an angel watching over me." Then he was asked to imagine the scene with an angel watching over him. He, as his current-age self was there, seeing his younger self hitting the concrete, and an angelic figure hovering above them. He said he saw a beam of light shining on his younger self and he knew he was going to be fine. Afterwards, he said he felt relief. Subsequently, he stopped having intrusive thoughts.

The book of norm

A strategy offered in Katz (2014) is the book of norm to help people see that what they may assume is logical or right may not be for another. In this metaphor, clients imagine that in the attic of their mind is a book of what is normal and expected. Imagine a thick leather-bound book resting on a pedestal with tissue-paper-thin pages. This book outlines all that should happen in life: how parents, friends, employers, romantic partners, drivers on the road, etc, should behave. It also states where one should be in life at every age: have this type of job, have this type of family, etc. It is the book of expectations (and judgments) for oneself and others. The problem is, others are not operating from the same book. They are literally not on the same page. It may seem incomprehensible that others make certain choices. But to them, it makes sense from their perspective. Even if they are operating from a limited point of view, they believe that they are right. They have their own motives and agendas, and are responding to their own holograms, fears, and desires. They are responding to their own book of norm.

Mentalization, observer vantage point, and multiple points of view

The strategies of observer vantage point and considering multiple points of view is consistent with Fonagy's work on mentalization (Fonagy, 2002). Mentalization is the ability to imagine a situation from another's perspective. Fonagy asserts that mentalization represents the epitome of human cognitive evolution and is the foundation of all effective psychotherapy. In holographic reprocessing, it is a process of stepping back from a situation, to embrace an observer vantage point to consider perspective. How else can we see this situation? What other meanings can we derive? Can we imagine it from another's point of view? It encourages a nonjudgmental attitude, curiosity, and inquisitiveness. Even if the perspectives or possible meanings that a therapist or client poses are not accurate, it helps to consider the possibility that there could be another way to see it. The possibility of a different perspective is usually sufficient to shift a tightly held belief. This is important to note for therapists, to allow themselves to consider possibilities without asserting that it is absolutely accurate, or even necessarily probable. The point is to put a crack in a cemented belief that is keeping a client stuck. It creates room for the client to release a personalization and consider that there may be more to the story.

In summary,

- The **observer vantage point** (as if an eagle observing from above) allows people to see all the people in the scene for a broader and more comprehensive perception compared to the **field vantage point** as if re-experiencing the event (e.g., field mouse)
- **Multiple truths** help people to see the same scene from different viewpoints (e.g., their agenda and motives)
- **Age comparison** facilitates understanding by considering the perspective of people at younger ages (e.g., self as young and innocent, or others who were either young themselves or old enough to know better)
- **Hindsight advantage** shifts fear in the field vantage point, by already knowing the outcome
- **Book of norm** helps people consider that they cannot assume what they think is right or reasonable is what others will think

Meaning-making: Reframes and meta-reframes

A meta-reframe is a holistic reappraisal at a broad level that changes the understanding of all layers below the layer of the reframe. The broader and more comprehensive the reframe, the more layers are reappraised. A meta-reframe is a comprehensive explanation that encompasses all other explanations to a broad enough extent that it provides a context for positive factors such as forgiveness, compassion, and gratitude.

Case example: Whale-watching trip

Anna and her 6-year-old son boarded a vessel to go whale watching. They sat next to another mom and her daughter. The children started to play. Once out on the water, another girl wandered over and started to play with them as well. They asked to go up on the deck and the moms agreed they could play upstairs. Soon, the little boy went back to his mom looking upset. He said they didn't want to play with him anymore. Upon further inquiry, it was the second little girl who said something unkind and told him to go away. Anna reframed the situation, and said it gave them an opportunity to focus on looking for whales and dolphins.

The girls came over to where Anna and her son were looking for whales. Her son started playing with them again. However, soon he returned to

Anna with dirt on his shirt. He said the second girl pushed him and told him he couldn't play with them anymore. Although Anna and her son saw a whale and lots of dolphins, she could tell he was still hurt by their interaction.

Then it was time to disembark. Anna saw the second girl's mother call to her. She was busy being very attentive to a disabled boy who appeared to be her son (the second girl's brother). The mom and boy carefully disembarked with the second girl walking alone behind her family. Anna wanted to help her son see the situation in a new way where he could understand the greater context, where he could see that there was possibly another explanation to the girl's behavior. She explained that maybe the little girl wanted to play with the first girl all to herself without having to share the attention with another boy because maybe what she really wanted is more time with her mother without having to share her attention with her brother.

Concerned that a 6-year-old may not fully understand, she asked if that made sense to him. He said, "Yes mama, I understand, she just wasn't being loved enough."

Meta-reframes

A meta-reframe is a comprehensive explanation, or a broader whole, that encompasses all other wholes and subsumes all other explanations. It is a way of understanding an individual, situation, or event with sufficient perspective to see contextual and relational variables. By using the observer vantage point, the personalization of the experience is removed, thus freeing the individual from being overly influenced by one's own emotional reactions. From this vantage point, new explanations and understandings can emerge. In contrast to a reframe which is designed to re-conceptualize an event, thought, or situation, a meta-reframe considers contextual factors, multiple points of view, and a broad framework for explaining and understanding a situation, relationship, or event. It considers multiple truths, or layers of truths in a situation and a broader context or perspective incorporating all other perspectives below it. A meta-reframe alters the understanding of multiple layers all at once.

In the example above, the reframe offered was to look on the bright side of a situation—seeing the opportunity in an apparently bad situation. Anna said, not playing with the girls was an opportunity to look for whales. This is a classic type of reframe—e.g., "making lemonade out of lemons." It was helpful, but it didn't answer *why* this happened or completely release the personalization. Even if the boy shifted his attention to the whales, he still may wonder why the second little girl didn't like him. It could potentially have an influence on his self-perception and willingness to engage in future similar situations. However, the meta-reframe removes the personalization and allows for a broader more comprehensive explanation. In fact, instead of him wondering about his own likability, he left the situation with an increased understanding for the very person who was being mean to him! Instead of closing his heart with anger and hurt, he opened his heart with compassion.

In summary, classic reframes are ways to look at the bright side of things, or thinking about a potential positive way to look at a situation. Reframing puts a new frame on a situation giving it a positive twist and more uplifting interpretation. However, a meta-reframe considers context, and thereby broadens one's perspective resulting in altering the understanding of a situation or event. It considers the person in context, including what others may be feeling or thinking. This draws upon mentalization skills and considering multiple truths. How could the situation make sense from other people's points of view or possibilities of other outcomes? It is a process of turning the tissue box around, considering all sides, stepping back as an eagle-observer and thinking of ways it can all make sense.

Sometimes clinicians worry if they are doing meta-reframes right, or are not sure if their explanation is accurate. This is not necessarily about being accurate, but rather about opening possibilities for a new way to make sense of a situation. It creates cognitive room to consider alternate explanations and maybe a more palatable way to hold a situation, especially for those situations that cannot be altered or changed. How else can a negative situation be interpreted?

More case examples:

1   A veteran was grieving the loss of her military career, thinking she would have been retired by now. She blamed her sexual trauma experience for cutting her desired military career short. However, she shifted to gratitude when she realized that if she stayed in the military, she wouldn't have met her current partner. She also described herself as an innocent lamb who was naïve and vulnerable. She most likely would have been sent to the Vietnam War and when considering that path not traveled, she concluded that the sexual trauma probably saved her life.

2   A gay child suffered from a rejection hologram beginning with rejection from his parents. When considering an alternate reality, where if he was straight and accepted by his parents, he would have been indoctrinated into his parent's way of thinking. He said that would have stunted his growth, just like his younger sister who is suffering from anxiety, dependency, and immaturity for her age. He appreciated not being accepted into a club where he would not want to be a member. Not only did he have freedom of thought, he realized that he was able to evolve past his parents and their limited point of view. We discussed how children are meant to evolve past parents to evolve the species.

3   An adult with strong spiritual beliefs was searching for meaning after experiencing severe child abuse. She thought, how could this make sense? Why would I choose to be born into this terrible family? She blamed herself for having bad karma and maybe she deserved to suffer. She shifted when we considered, "Where would a light-being choose to shine her light?" She responded, "in the darkest places she could find." This gave her experience meaning consistent with her values and sense of purpose. She was able to send her young self love and compassion in her reprocessing imagery. She saw her experience as part of her dharma (purpose), and it was instrumental in her decision to open a series of homes for orphaned children in India.

4   An ex-convict was searching for self-esteem from a family who abused alcohol and were convicted for various crimes. He said, "I'm no-good just like my father and grandfather." We discussed a meta-reframe that he was such a loyal loving son! He mirrored their behavior which made them feel comfortable, rather than choosing a path that would be confrontational or threatening. He made choices out of his love and loyalty to them. But now as an adult, he is free to live consistent with his own beliefs and values. He said what he wanted to do was go back to school and become a social worker.

5   A woman during a rape, stopped resisting and gave up her will and her power. She blamed herself for giving up. She said she was weak and was disgusted with herself. We discussed the situation, and concluded that actually, this was a powerful choice. He was becoming more violent, and further resistance could have led to worse outcomes. We discussed that intuitively she knew what to do to get through it as best as she could. We concluded that she has excellent instincts, and this is powerful. She was and always will be powerful.

6   An adult was struggling with her self-esteem. She said as a child she believed she was not worthy, incapable, and stupid. She knew she was smart inside but went along with the belittlement from her parents. She was blaming herself and didn't understand why she would let them treat her that way. We discussed that she loved them and likely went along with it as a selfless loving act, to protect her insecure parents. She shifted from anger (from focusing on the injustice) and her own insecurities to seeing her parents' limitations and anxiety. She had compassion for her younger self. She knew she had evolved past her parents, was grateful for the sacrifices they made for her, but now she was ready to protect and nurture her younger self.

7   A woman was grieving a miscarriage, she realized that she has a special bond with her child. She'll always have this bond and didn't know she could love that deeply. The meta-reframe is that this child forever opened her heart.

Considerations for meta-reframes

The following is offered as some guidance for generating meta-reframes. It is not exhaustive or prescriptive, but rather suggestions to generate possibilities. Meta-reframes can also be encouraged by clients—what else could be a possible explanation or way to make sense of this? The challenge is to think of seeing the past from a larger perspective, other sides of the tissue box, what else could it mean?

Important note

Meta-reframes are not intended to make light of or minimize someone's experience. It is important to be sensitive when this is implemented to make sure people do not feel it is a flippant, discounting explanation as if to say, "Oh well, it could have been worse." It is important to fully validate and acknowledge one's experience before exploring another perspective. Be clear that this is meant to consider a less painful way to make sense of going through something significant. It is offered with compassion, never judgment.

Losses and regrets (e.g., "If only this didn't happen, I would be better off," or "If only I did this action, this event wouldn't have happened")

- First validate, acknowledge, understand.
- Then entertain the client's what-ifs. Maybe it would have been better, or maybe not.
- Consider it may or may not have been averted. If someone is motivated to do a crime, or are pre-meditating an action, they will look for an opportunity.
- It may have been worse. Violence increases with resistance and there is always the possibility that things could have been worse.
- Others were involved who contributed to making it happen. We don't know if things were different, that it would have been better.
- Consider any gains or benefits as a result of going through a trauma or loss.
- How could the loss motivate positive change? How could you honor the deceased? Share gratitude for the love they had or stay close to someone loved?

Grieving a poor outcome

- Acknowledge loss and then consider how it might have led to something else, perhaps helped them or served a bigger picture. How has that event led to being here now?

Judging self for choices, mistakes, or outcomes

- Consider what was influencing them at the time.
- Consider others involved (appropriate blame and releasing through poetic justice).
- Consider how the experience may be useful/motivating moving forward.
- If consistent with a client's beliefs, consider a spiritual perspective, a grand plan, or an unknown reason that may serve a higher purpose.

Meta-reframes vs cognitive restructuring

Cognitive restructuring confronts negative thoughts (e.g., I'm no good), problematic thinking (e.g., all or nothing, jumping to conclusions), dysfunctional beliefs (e.g., all men/women can't be trusted) by asking clients to consider evidence for or against the thoughts to evaluate if the thought is logical or true. The intent is to invalidate problematic thinking.

Holographic reprocessing is not about discounting a thought, but rather seeing it as a potentially understandable piece of a bigger picture by considering multiple perspectives or multiple truths. The observer vantage point not only helps clients see context for their emotional thoughts but also allows for broader understanding and thereby, a more comprehensive truth. Instead of focusing on specific thoughts, holographic reprocessing seeks to understand themes, patterns, and explanations beyond oneself. It also allows for a more compassionate perspective to consider other people's motives, or their attempts to try to fulfill their unmet needs, avoid their fears, and compensate for their perceived inadequacies. What holograms are they responding to?

Meta-reframes focus on potential meaning and new ways to make sense of a situation from viewing it from various perspectives. In this way, it is restructuring the whole picture. Whereas cognitive restructuring focuses upon language (thoughts), meta-reframes focus on images, sensations, and the skills of mentalization to imagine how and why others feel and act the way that they do.

Acceptance

Acceptance is the final stage of grief according to Elizabeth Kubler-Ross (1970). It is surrendering to what is and what was. It is incorporating a loss or trauma into one's new reality, adjusting to the new reality as it is. Acceptance does not mean agreeing with or that it is okay. Some things are never okay and some things are unforgivable. Acceptance does not minimize the loss or trauma, nor in any way is meant to diminish or discount it. It means coming to the here and now and choosing to live.

Linehan (1993) uses the term *radical acceptance* to mean coming to terms with what is. It is a radical shift that halts all of the would-haves and could-haves. No more if-only thinking. It just is. The past is over. However, while acceptance is an important part of healing, it is not necessarily easy. Every fiber in one's body may be fighting to say no, no, no, this can't be. People can be stuck in their grief and non-acceptance for years. But once people can receive acceptance, there is a wonderful freedom from the struggle of grief, shock, anger, and non-acceptance. It is the release of all the upset that weighs people down. It frees people to be in the present and open to their future.

The blue pen

A metaphor to aid in radical acceptance is the blue pen exercise (Katz, 2014). A client is offered to hold a blue pen and asked, what color pen do they have? They respond that they have a blue pen. Do they have this red one? Or this yellow one? No, what they have is blue. Regardless if a client likes or doesn't like it, or feels they deserve or should have had a red one, it does not change what is in their hand. It is still blue. They may be angry, resentful, and think it is unfair that they have a blue one. Maybe the client wants to stomp on it, yell at it, cry, or scream. Regardless of what they think or feel, it is still blue. Waking up daily, spending months or years wanting the past to be different than it is, is as futile as wanting the pen to be anything other than what it is. It is blue. And the past is the past.

But once someone is able to take ownership of their blue pen, and come to terms with the reality of what was and what is, they can embrace the power of the blue pen. The power is in radical acceptance, as it frees up all the expended energy on wanting a different pen. The power is accepting the blue pen and thinking about what is important now, and what do they want to create in the rest of the life that they have.

Disengaging from the past

For some, the word acceptance is offensive, as the events from the past are gravely unacceptable. It is advised not to try to argue the benefits or meaning of acceptance. Instead, a more neutral and accurate word is to *disengage* from the past. This is a critical step between suffering and coming to terms with what is. The step is to disengage.

Poetic justice—disengaging from anger

As mentioned previously, anger and resentment, especially from an injustice, can disrupt healing. How does one heal from a horrible event inflicted from someone when there was no closure, no justice, and no consequences for the perpetrator? It's a conundrum: anger can be both completely justified and can completely derail one's health and well-being. While people have a right to be angry, don't they also deserve to be happy and free? The strategy of poetic justice (Katz, 2014) is offered as a way to release the toxic effects of anger without negating the issue of having a lack of justice or closure.

People tend to be consistent: If they have done something bad in the past, chances are that they will repeat that behavior—and they will suffer the natural consequences when they do. We may not know when or how this will occur, but poetic justice means that everyone will get their consequences. Poetic justice is the belief that **somehow, someway, somewhere, people reap the consequences of their behaviors.** People know when they have committed a crime, assaulted another, or engaged in immoral behavior. They know what they did, even if they pretend they don't, or deny it… even if they convince others that they didn't do it, even if they try to blame their victims, they still know that they did it. Their malicious actions were intentional. If they have a conscience, they may feel guilt, regret, moral injury, or shame. Maybe they worry about being caught or publicly humiliated. If they don't care, then likely they will continue to behave in ways that will lead to natural consequences. It will eventually catch up to them. Perhaps there will be spiritual justice after they leave this life. Poetic justice means what happens to others is their problem, their journey, and their own issue.

Therapists can say, "Imagine washing your hands of the past, and freeing your mind. Know, that somehow, someway, justice will be served. Freedom is disengaging from thoughts, emotions, or energetic connections to the negative past. Like releasing a balloon, watch it float away."

Shrinking machine

In this strategy, the client imagines a machine of their design to shrink something that is scary, large, loud, intimidating, and threatening to something very small. For example, shrinking a dominating abusive person into a tiny person waving their arms and squeaking, takes the power from them. If it is comical, that is a bonus. One client imagined shrinking her abusive boyfriend and imagined him driving away in his tiny car. The client can create and direct the imagery with the intention to shrink the fear and regain empowerment.

Catcher's mitt

This strategy is used to create a barrier from receiving abuse or negativity from another person, and then bounce it back to the owner, or dispose of it such as throwing it in a garbage can. This is a guided imagery procedure where the client imagines seeing the person spewing negativity (silently) and dark smoke is coming from their mouth. Then the person turns toward them and spews the smoke, but the client holds up a large catcher's mitt and the smoke is sucked up by the mitt. The client rolls it into a ball and tosses it back. For example, Eric realized his anxiety, paranoia, and depression was inherited from his father because of his father's history of trauma. He imagined him as his current-age self with his younger self by his side tossing his father's negativity back to him. He said, "This is yours, not mine."

It takes a thief for a theft (putting blame where blame is due)

It takes a thief for a theft to occur. As discussed in Chapter 9, this metaphor puts blame on a perpetrator not a victim. The person who knowingly engages in behaviors that are wrong is the one who is at fault for the abuse. A wallet cannot thieve itself. This concept requires stepping outside of one's experience to consider the thief, their motive, and intention independent from the victim.

Chapter summary

This chapter covers ways to consider context for gaining perspective, consider one's experience from a different vantage point, and perhaps consider a new meaning or way to understand past experiences. Then it offers several strategies to disengage and release connection to anger, blame, or ownership of something that is not theirs.

- Observer vantage point (eagle) helps broaden one's view of the past or situation, whereas the field vantage point (field mouse) only sees events from the perspective of being in it
- Multiple points of view sees other points of view (their motives, agendas, perspective) without refuting one's own
  - Age comparison and hindsight advantage facilitate reviewing the past with new knowledge that changes how they view it
  - Book of norm—what is written in one's book of assumptions can be very different for someone else's book
- Meta-reframes consider a broad comprehensive explanation for an event that changes how one thinks about their past
- Acceptance and disengaging helps release attachment to the past
  - Blue pen—it is blue and we can't change the past or the color of the pen
  - Poetic justice—that people reap natural consequences of their own behaviors

- **Shrinking machine**—reduces something fearful to something small and comical
- **Catcher's mitt**—creates a barrier to no longer receive negativity or verbal abuse from someone. It is empowering as well as disengaging from an old pattern
- **It takes a thief**—lets other people be responsible for their own actions, and releases responsibility for something that belongs to another

Chapter 11

Imagery reprocessing

This chapter presents the technique of imagery reprocessing. It outlines the preparation and steps for implementing the technique. Clients think about who they want to visit. As their current-age self, what would they like to say and what would they like to do, if they could meet their younger self? It also discusses the differences between rescripting (changing imagery) and reprocessing (offering a healing message). A rescripting component can be added to one's imagery, but ultimately, the imagery is to end with reprocessing where the current-age self offers compassion or understanding to their younger self. Various versions are offered for releasing grief, fear, and self-blame.

Case example: What about me?

Heather a 26-year-old Asian-American woman said the reason she was coming for therapy was because she has been very irritated and angry with her boyfriend. She was not sure if she should stay with him. There was an incident where her boyfriend was not paying attention to her, and she had an angry outburst. He was on the phone with a female co-worker. They were laughing and talking. She felt left out, and started dancing to get his attention; when he asked her to stop, she was enraged. She screamed at him for being selfish and inconsiderate. After the first session, it was clear that her feelings of anger were related to something deeper in her past.

Heather appeared particularly uncomfortable in session. She described herself as shy and feeling self-conscious. She had difficulty expressing herself. She waited for me to ask her questions. Even if the questions were open-ended, she would give very brief responses. I asked if we could do a time-line of her life, thinking it could be an in-road to discussing her feelings about her past. She agreed. She said the first major event occurred when she was four. She stated she had an ear infection and was hospitalized. Her parents couldn't stand to see her hospitalized so they didn't visit her. She

DOI: 10.4324/9781003223429-13

remembered feeling all alone in the hospital. She still is angry that her parents left her there.

Then she told me about how her family had to move every few years because of her father's career. She reported how she always tried to "fit in" with the other children. However, she stated she was shy and was teased and picked on. We discussed how this was scary and lonely. She so much wanted to be accepted and liked. She remembered going to a new high school and one of the most popular senior boys asked her out on a date. He drove her to the countryside where he sexually assaulted her in the back of his truck. After that incident, she started using alcohol and drugs. She didn't tell anyone about the rape. Her parents felt she was "out of control" so they sent her to a boarding school for difficult teenagers. This was very restrictive and not once did anyone ask her to share her feelings.

We mapped her experiential hologram of neglect. She could see the pattern where she felt alone, and her feelings were ignored. She could see how her anger outbursts were her way of getting attention, trying to get people to listen to her. She was connecting the events of her life. She also started implementing slow deep breathing, and increasing awareness of her feelings in her body.

We discussed how she wanted to give herself as a little girl a hug. We did a visualization where she went to her little girl self and told her that she listens to everything she has to say. I facilitated a dialogue, reinforcing that she is always there for her and she will never be left alone again. I taught her how she could hug herself by crossing her arms so that her right-hand rests on her left shoulder and her left-hand rests on her right shoulder. She reported that this felt good.

In the next session, she stated that she went to her old school yard and imagined seeing herself getting teased by the other children. She spontaneously created a visualization where her adult self-comforted her younger self. She was proud of her mastery of this technique and stated it made her feel much better. She also reported a recalled memory of herself at age four having a temper tantrum on the floor at an airport. She remembered kicking and screaming at the top of her lungs. She remembered the inside of her ear was extremely painful. She was trying to express her discomfort to her parents and they ignored her. She had the temper tantrum to get their attention. Since they did not take her to the doctor to get her ear checked, the problem developed into a life-threatening infection for which she was hospitalized. Again, we did a comforting visualization at her request.

She said she was ready to visit her younger self during the rape. What she experienced was a perception of the event from a new perspective. She saw a young girl struggling for attention. She saw a young girl who was scared and confused. She saw that she had no idea what was really happening and part of her even thought she was doing the right thing. She saw a girl that was naïve and most importantly she saw a girl that was innocent. She talked to the girl and told her she was innocent (e.g., it was not her fault). She held her and cried and declared that she would protect her.

After the treatment, she stated that she felt a release of tension from her stomach. She said she felt "lighter and more at peace." Heather had a very positive response to this treatment.

She stopped having the angry outbursts when she realized why she got angry (feeling ignored/neglected). She was ready to learn more effective ways to meet these needs. She continued to work on affect regulation skills and improving her communication skills.

Imagery reprocessing

Imagery reprocessing is a procedure where one's current-age self imagines visiting their younger self or someone deceased. This occurs after working on understanding the past with context such as mapping one's experiential hologram and considering context from the observer vantage point and perhaps meta-reframes. Heather had a neglect hologram with multiple examples re-enacting what she went through and how it made her feel. She was able to see her pattern and how that led to being vulnerable to the attention and (false) affections of a popular senior in high school. When she visited her younger self in the imagery, she finally knew at a deep level that she was innocent, it was not her fault, and she vowed to take care of her younger (and current-age) self from now on.

Imagery reprocessing can be tailored to the needs of the client. Some will only do it once, and others like Heather wanted to do it multiple times, each time deepening her healing process. The content can also be tailored depending on the need of the client (e.g., secondary to a moral injury, completing grief, or offering understanding, reassurance, safety, or love to an abused younger self).

In the following example (Katz, 2005), 70-year-old Edward completed reprocessing of being gang-raped while serving in the military. He stated, "I was an 18-year-old kid and now looking back at it as a man, I realize that the 18-year-old really couldn't have done anything about it. Looking at it as a man, I can see that the kid was really helpless... He couldn't have fought them off. It wasn't his fault." When reprocessing was first offered to Edward, he was hesitant but then was surprised that it "wasn't that bad." He did it a second time and said he felt a tremendous relief including feeling less ashamed and less blamed.

In both of these examples (Heather and Edward), offering self-compassion through reprocessing helped them heal. This is consistent with Bhuptani and Messman's (2022) research demonstrating that targeting self-compassion to reduce rape-related shame, subsequently facilitated reductions in PTSD and depression symptoms.

In reprocessing, fear and arousal are intentionally minimized by using the observer vantage point. This helps people remain aware of their current-age self (who is safe and in the present moment) while imagining viewing the younger self without feeling as if they are re-experiencing events from the past. This helps to reduce stress and to make it a comfortable experience.

Objectives of reprocessing

As outlined in Katz (2005) there are several objectives that can be addressed through reprocessing.

Delivering communications

Reprocessing is an opportunity to imagine delivering a communication to someone where it feels unresolved. This could be to someone who died, or to one's parents or other family member, or to their younger self. These communications are designed to be tender and compassionate (i.e., saying good-bye, or giving and receiving an apology, or telling one's younger self, they did a good job, it's not their fault, or simply offering them love). The idea is to facilitate closure by delivering a communication. The client can imagine the recipient of the communication responding in an appropriate manner. This is not designed to communicate hostilities or threats to a perpetrator. If this is what the client desires, then further work on anger and resentment would be helpful (not something done in imagery).

Gaining insight or awareness

Even after considering context and meta-reframes, sometimes in imagery reprocessing, clients will spontaneously understand something in a new way. Sometimes clients report an insight, new memory, or more compassion for their younger self.

Increasing a sense of power

Sometimes clients need to reclaim their sense of power by imagining being in an empowering role. In an earlier example of Edward who was gang-raped, he wanted to imagine rescripting the event and fighting off the assailants. He imagined him as his current age alongside his younger self successfully fighting them off. Sometimes clients find it easier to feel empowered when they are fighting for someone else such as their younger self. Another example is having the current-age self rescuing one's younger self. This helps them experience a sense of power and reinforces that they do have the ability to be powerful in difficult situations.

Note: this is an example of rescripting or imagining a different ending; the reprocessing part would be communicating something healing to the younger self.

Returning to safety

Reoccurring fear of being unsafe can be addressed through reprocessing. This can be achieved by having the client reassure and comfort the younger self. Using the hindsight advantage, clients can reassure the younger self that they will make it through a difficult situation. The current-age self goes back to the younger self and tells them they are going to be okay.

Offering self-forgiveness, comfort, understanding, and/or reassurance

Reprocessing facilitates self-acceptance and self-forgiveness. This includes offering comfort to a younger self in distress, reassurance that they are going to be okay, or offering understanding from the perspective of their current age. Commonly, it entails communicating that what happened was not the younger self's fault; they are not alone; and they will be taken care of from now on.

Releasing grief and/or negative emotions

Reprocessing is about releasing untruths about oneself or others, imagining releasing the souls of someone deceased, releasing negative emotions that no longer serve the client, seeking closure, releasing anger, hurt, or anything that was weighing down the client regarding the past. In the imagery, clients can release the negativity and feel relief.

Controversy of forgiving perpetrators

Forgiveness can be a tricky topic, as some people believe that the only way to heal is to forgive their perpetrator. This may be a pathway for some, but it can also put an extra burden on clients. Forgiveness of a perpetrator may or may not ever occur for some clients, nor is it necessary to heal. As one client stated, "some things are unforgivable." Others may say they forgive the sinner not the sin, and some will say that the forgiveness helps them, not the perpetrator. However, these are delicate topics and highly individualized.

One way to address this is to ask to wait until the client thoroughly processes their own feelings (e.g., focus the reprocessing on the needs of the younger self in the scene). Premature forgiveness of a perpetrator can lead to resentment, further incomplete feelings, guilt, and self-blame. When people are pressured to focus on forgiving their perpetrators, they run the risk of continuing a pattern where they are supposed to attend to other people's needs (including making other people feel more comfortable) while deep inside feel their hurt is minimized and their own needs are being ignored.

A more reasonable goal is to focus on supporting clients to feel empowered and safe, distant, and protected from their perpetrator. This is where poetic justice can be useful. The client can release their connection with the perpetrator and let the perpetrator incur their own natural consequences. This frees the client not to think about them at all, neither for forgiveness or revenge. What happens to the perpetrator is the perpetrator's problem, allowing the client to disengage and focus on their own healing. The goal is to disengage, not necessarily accept or forgive, but rather release any ties (cognitive and emotionally) that bind a person to a perpetrator or to the trauma.

Ironically, once people work on their own healing, and release themselves from the wrongs of the past, then they may (or may not) be in a place to consider compassion for someone who hurt others. But this is after allowing the victim to feel fully acknowledged, understood, and helped, and again, forgiveness is not necessary for healing, but disengaging is.

Imagery reprocessing techniques

Imagery reprocessing is where a client is guided to imagine a scene before or usually after a traumatic incident. The client remains their current age and can interact with the characters in the scene but most importantly delivers a message to one's younger self.

Writing a letter

Writing letters such as to someone deceased or to one's younger self is a way to help clients think about what they want to communicate before engaging in imagery. It is a process of putting their thoughts and feelings into words. If shared with the therapist, it allows the therapist to gauge the client's perceptions. Is the communication supportive, healing, and hopeful? Or is the client warning, or blaming the younger self? If the therapist has any concerns about a client engaging in imagery reprocessing, letter writing is a great step. It also helps clients say everything they want to say, which in itself can be a relief. If doing imagery reprocessing in a group, letter writing is recommended to ensure the readiness and safety of everyone in the group.

Instructions for writing a letter to one's young self

"Take a few moments and imagine you could visit your younger self. What would you like to say? What does your younger self need to hear from you?

What can you give your younger self that would provide comfort, love, and safety? What would you like to do?"

Some people want to give their younger self a hug and let them know it wasn't their fault, they are good and worthy, and from now on, they will be protected, listened to, and cared for. The idea is that the client as their current-age self, knowing what they know now, has an opportunity to right something from their past. The current self can offer the caring, understanding, encouragement, or safety that the younger self didn't get.

Note: Younger self can be any age younger than the client is now—from childhood to adulthood, any younger self that could benefit from a letter from the current-age self. They may want to write more than one letter, such as one to the childhood self and one to a younger self in adulthood.

Instructions for implementing reprocessing

The work of mapping experiential holograms, considering context, should give both the therapist and client a clear sense of the issue that is in need of addressing. In preparation, the client may want to answer the following questions:

1   What is your core violation (to the best of your ability)? For example: being neglected, rejected, betrayed, or endangered; survivor of a threatening experience; unresolved grief; unresolved guilt.
2   What was your unmet need? For example: lack of attention, acceptance, loyalty, freedom, safety, validation, forgiveness.
3   What would you like to tell your younger self? What does your younger self need from you? For example: "it's not your fault," "you are not alone," "you did a good job," etc. If the reprocessing is to complete an interaction with someone who has deceased, then the question is: What would you like to tell the other person? Is there something you want them to know?

Question: Why don't we revisit trauma in reprocessing?

Imagery reprocessing is not a desensitization procedure. It is not meant to trigger or traumatize clients, but rather it is a gentle imagery exercise designed to help clients connect with their younger self. This can be emotional, but not frightening. It's important for clients to be reassured that they are in control of their imagery. It is helpful to think about what they want to say/do before the imagery, and they can stop or redirect the imagery at any time.

Preparation for reprocessing (questions for clients):

1   Think of an age of your younger self that you would like to visit. Where is your younger self? What is your younger self doing?

2   What would you want to say to your younger self? What do you think your younger self would like to hear from you? (e.g., "You're going to be ok," "I'll take care of you," "It wasn't your fault," "You did the best you could," "I love you!")
3   What would you want to do for your younger self? What do you think your younger self would like you to do? (e.g., "Go to a garden," "Keep her in my heart," "Give him a hug")

Important note

Do not revisit images of trauma as this is not a desensitization procedure.

Preparing for reprocessing

As outlined in Katz (2005), imagery reprocessing is prepared for by: 1) Asking for permission; 2) contextualizing the scene; 3) training on recalling a memory from the observer vantage point; 4) ensuring safety and relaxation.

Step 1: Informed consent

As with any new procedure, informed consent is the first step. This includes explaining the rationale and the procedure itself, and giving the client an opportunity to ask questions. A therapist can also offer an alternative if the client has any reservations. Clients should feel comfortable and freely choose to proceed.

Presenting rationale for the procedure

This is usually a brief statement explaining that imagery reprocessing is a guided imagery exercise where they as their current-age self visits their younger self to offer a healing communication. It is designed as a way to get closure with the past.

Explaining the steps of the procedure

The therapist briefly explains the processes of: relaxation, guided imagery, slowly approaching the scene, using the observer vantage point, and imagery reprocessing. Therapists ask if clients have questions about the procedure.

Reassuring clients

Reassure clients that they will not be re-experiencing their trauma. They are not to revisit images of trauma, but rather pick a time when they can visit their younger self in a safe place. If at any time in the procedure they feel uncomfortable, they can switch to a positive image such as being in a garden. They can stop at any time. If clients are hesitant or nervous about doing the exercise, they might opt to just do the relaxation and guided imagery parts of the procedure. The therapist can reassure clients that they always have control—they can communicate how they are feeling, change the imagery, or stop the procedure at any time.

Step 2: Choosing a scene for reprocessing

Discuss which age younger self the client would like to visit. What led up to the event and what happened afterwards? The therapist can inquire about how old the younger self is, what are they doing, and anything else about the context of the younger self.

If visiting a younger self is too triggering of trauma, then they can choose a younger self at a different, less threatening time. The same experiential hologram will likely be evident, embodying the same core violation and personalization. Reprocessing a current situation may be effective to break the holographic cycle, if the client is able to link the current situation to a pattern of similar experiences. Maybe after having a comfortable experience, they may be ready to reprocess with a younger self who had been through a more difficult experience. Some clients, as in the example of Heather, find benefit in reprocessing several events including specific traumas from adulthood as well as from childhood.

This is also the time to make sure that the introductory imagery to assist with relaxation is safe and neutral. If walking through a forest or country road is a trauma-trigger, then use an alternative nature scene such as the beach.

Step 3: Training in the observer vantage point

Exercise: Recalling last night's dinner

The following exercise teaches clients the difference between engaging in imagery from the two vantage points. When recalling a memory from the field vantage point it is as if re-experiencing the event, as if it is happening right now. However, recalling a memory from the observer vantage point, if observing it, is like watching it from afar. The following is an exercise to understand recalling an event from the two vantage points.

1   First identify what you had for dinner last night (or another recent meal).
2   Then take a cleansing breath to relax. Gently close your eyes and recall last night's dinner as you were reliving the experience of eating dinner. Imagine yourself taking a bite of the food... Make the image as vivid as you can... and then open your eyes.

3   Now, let's do the exercise again. But this time recall the event as if you are observing yourself eating dinner. Take a cleansing breath to relax. Gently close your eyes and recall last night's dinner as if you are observing yourself eating dinner. Imagine watching yourself take a bite of the food... Make the image as vivid as you can... and then open your eyes.

4   What did you experience? What did you notice the first time? How about the second time? Which time did the food taste better? Did you notice things about the space around you and how you looked?

Recollection from the field vantage should be associated with more emotions, tasting the food, and remembering the experience of eating. However, the observer vantage point should be associated with observing the event, seeing oneself, what else was in the room, and maybe judging what one looked like while eating, but not actually tasting the food. Consistent with the McIsaac and Eich (2002, 2004) studies, the field vantage point was more emotional and experiential while the observer vantage point gave the experience context. In imagery reprocessing, we use the observer vantage point. Instead of imaging being one's younger self, clients imagine observing one's younger self through the eyes of their current self.

Step 4: Ensuring safety and relaxation

Imagery reprocessing begins with grounding and relaxation. This helps facilitate the client's ability to concentrate and stay connected with the imagery. Anxiety disrupts the process and activates dysregulation. Relaxation can be as simple as practicing slow deep breathing, or a body scan. Depending on the client needs, basic relaxation can be extended, shortened, modified, or even skipped.

Basic relaxation script

"Let's start with a signal breath, deep breath in through the nose, hold it at the top... then exhale through the mouth... signaling the body it's time to relax. And again, deep breath in... hold it... and then exhale. And as you exhale feel your shoulders release, letting go of any tension in your body. Breathing a bit slower and deeper, releasing with each exhale through your shoulders and chest. Exhaling all the way to the ground. Maybe roll your shoulders and release your neck... letting your arms rest comfortably in your lap. Feeling the weight of your body sitting in the chair, your back is supported, your feet are on the ground feeling supported, and your whole body can just melt into the chair."

Optional comments

Some clients might benefit from reassuring words from the therapist. This is entirely optional and not necessary for the practice of reprocessing.

"Now you are ready for deep healing... know that your life experiences have led you to this point and have prepared you for this exercise. You are ready to complete the past, make things right, so you can live a satisfying and happy life. You have the wisdom and perspective of your current age to help you understand and appreciate life in new and meaningful ways."

The goal for this section is for the client to hear positive, encouraging words. It further relaxes clients and helps them maintain the vantage point of their current age.

Next, guided imagery is introduced with attention to all the senses. This is to activate imagery and the experiential system.

"Imagine you are walking down a dirt path into a forest. It's a beautiful sunny day with a bright blue sky. You can feel the warmth of the sun on your skin. Already, you feel more relaxed as you walk along the path. You look around and see tiny pink and yellow wild flowers against a backdrop of majestic pine trees. You can smell the distinct scent of pine in the air. A songbird flies by and you can hear other birds chirping in the distance. You take in a deep breath of the fresh air, so nice and clean and refreshing. You continue walking on the path and can feel some dried leaves crunching underneath your shoes. It's a beautiful day and you are taking in all the beauty of nature."

The goal for this section is to introduce imagery. All the senses are mentioned, which helps deepen client engagement. The imagery is typically walking down a path either on a country road or into a forest. The idea of walking "deeper into the forest" is a metaphor for going deeper into a relaxed state. If the client was traumatized in the forest, then of course, you would change the imagery so that the client would feel safe and relaxed. Again, this can be extended or shortened depending on the needs of the client.

"On a scale from 1 to 10, where 10 is tense and 1 is very relaxed, where would you be on this scale? (After whatever answer is given, say: "Good," or "Excellent, keep breathing...")

If clients are still tense or if they report a number higher than 6, then it is recommended to continue with relaxation. The goal of this section is to check the level of relaxation for your client. If the client **is not ready** to do a reprocessing procedure, then continue with guided imagery such as:

"Up ahead you see a grass clearing. The grass is deep green and soft. There is a big boulder resting on the bank of a stream. You walk up to the boulder and see that it is smooth and shaped in such a way that it would be very comfortable to lean against it. Imagine sitting on the grass against the boulder, basking in the sun, breathing in the fresh, clean air, listening to the sounds of the stream. Taking your time to relax and enjoy this moment in nature. On the scale of 1 to 10, where might you be?"

If the client is ready to continue, then continue.

Step 5: Imagery reprocessing

If the client **is ready** to do a reprocessing procedure, then continue with the following:

"Far in the distance you can see where your younger self is. It is foggy but you can see that it is a place that looks familiar. Are you ready to move forward? (Client nods yes) Good. Now, imagine we are approaching the place where your younger self is. The image is still a little hazy. You are you, at your current age, with all the awareness and wisdom that you have."

If concerned about their level of relaxation you can ask, "where might you be on the 1 to 10 scale?" Check to see if the client is ready to approach the scene. The approach is slow, keeping the image distant, hazy, and small. If the client is able to maintain relaxation, then guide the client closer to the image and proceed with reprocessing. Based on the information the client has shared in previous sessions, the therapist can ask questions to help the client set up the characters in the scene. The therapist might ask the client to describe the scene. The scene should not be an image of trauma but rather just before or after.

"Imagine you are in front of the place where your younger self is. Breathe... and when you are ready, enter the place. Look around and find your younger self. What does your younger self look like? What is your younger self doing? You can approach and have a conversation. What would you like to say to your younger version of yourself? (*Pause...*) What would you like to do? (*Pause...*) Anything else? (*Pause...*) Are you ready to complete your visit?"

If the client is complete with the scene, they can imagine leaving the younger self in the original context or move the younger self to another place. Some clients prefer to imagine holding the younger version of the self in their hearts, some prefer to keep them in their house, and others prefer to remove them from the house and take them to a safe place such as to a beautiful garden. The therapist asks what the client wants and lets the client guide the imagery.

Afterwards, the client is instructed to walk back through the forest while the therapist facilitates the client's awareness of the here and now. After completing either the imagery or the reprocessing then the therapist closes the procedure with the following:

> "Imagine walking back through the forest. Everything appears to be a bit brighter, crisper, and clearer. You look around and see the beautiful trees and flowers. Breathing in the fresh air. Coming up (tone of voice goes up) through the forest. Now bring your awareness to where you are in this room, sitting on this chair. Feeling your toes… When you are ready, slowly open your eyes. Stretching and yawning…"

Allow clients time to adjust by sitting with a few moments of silence.

Step 6: Debriefing with the client

After the procedure, clients may need a few minutes to adjust. They may want to discuss what their experience was like, how they are feeling, or may just want a few moments of silence. The therapist can answer questions and help clients stay connected to their experience or simply sit with their feelings. Some clients go through a period of time where they work on incorporating the experience. It is helpful if therapists encourage their clients to take care of themselves in the weeks following reprocessing. Clients may recall certain memories, or may have unusual dreams, or insights. They may want to discuss their experience over several sessions. Other clients report that the exercise itself brought them closure and seem to have immediate acceptance of the new reprocessed perception.

Ensuring minimal arousal during exposure

Imagery reprocessing is designed to be safe with minimal arousal. While it may be emotional, and the client may be tearful, it should not lead to re-experiencing trauma or intense fear. Therapists can monitor client reactions to ensure therapeutic emotional distance, a sense of safety, and maintaining relaxation during the exercise. As outlined in Katz (2005) several strategies can help maintain minimal arousal.

Maintaining an observer vantage point

The observer vantage point helps clients focus on what happened in a situation rather than shifting to re-experiencing trauma. Clients are reminded that they are their current age looking back on the situation. This creates emotional distance and helps maintain the observer vantage point. The current age also helps anchor clients in the here and now. Refer to the younger self in the third person such as, "What is he/she/they doing?"

Monitor if the client speaks about the younger self in the first person such as "I am doing this." If so, gently remind the client that they are their current age meeting their younger self and the therapist uses the third-person language to assist. If the client doesn't shift, they are at risk of re-experiencing trauma and may need to be redirected out of the imagery.

Hindsight advantage

As previously discussed, the hindsight advantage is knowing the outcome of the situation. The fact that a client is sitting in the therapist's office means that they are "okay" and they have survived. This is particularly helpful when reprocessing events where there was a threat of danger.

Communicating with clients

During the reprocessing, it is okay for therapists to communicate with their clients. This does not mean engaging in a full conversation, because that would interfere with the procedure. Rather, the therapist can ask questions requiring short responses to keep in communication. For example, a therapist might ask clients how relaxed they are on a scale of 1 to 10, where 10 is tense and 1 is very relaxed. Or a question such as, "Are you ready to proceed?" The therapist reassures clients through the process, "You're doing great" or "good." It may seem counter-intuitive to disrupt a client by asking a question. Indeed, it may cause a momentary disruption, but once the client re-engages, it can actually deepen the connection. Alternatively, the therapist can ask the client to nod their head if they are okay or if they are ready to continue.

Observing and monitoring clients

Therapists can observe the body language of their clients to monitor if they seem uncomfortable or tense. If this is during the initial relaxation phase, the therapist could say, "... and breathe" or "with this next exhale, release your shoulders, and drop into a place of ease." "Feel your feet on the ground, anchoring you as your current-age self to the here and now."

If concerned, the therapist can ask if they are okay. Sometimes clients will furrow their eyebrows or show emotion in their faces. Not all intense emotions are signs to intervene. It could be a sign they are deeply engaged. Many clients cry during this procedure. Imagery reprocessing, can be and often is, an emotional experience, but not a traumatic one.

If clients are struggling, therapists can slow down the procedure, take more time relaxing, or stop. If a client cannot maintain the observer vantage point, even with therapist support, they may not be ready to engage in reprocessing, or perhaps the chosen scene was too upsetting.

Redirecting the imagery

If clients are with their younger self and they start to feel upset or unsafe, the therapist can ask, if they are okay, or what they need? Therapists can ask if the client would like to do something, or take their younger self to a different place. The therapist remains calm and conveys confidence. Therapist attunement with their client, helps emotionally regulate the client. If desired, the therapist can help the client redirect the imagery to a safe place (e.g., a garden) reassuring them that they are safe now.

Getting assistance

If a client is struggling in the imagery the therapist can ask if they would like anyone to join them in the imagery. It could be a friend/family member, someone from the spirit world, a pet, or a mythical or religious figure. One client wanted Archangel Michael to help protect her. Consistent with de Rios (1997) work on magical realism, clients can use culturally or religiously relevant images to assist them.

Changing attributes

Changing attributes of an image can help increase emotional distance. Highly emotional images are big, loud, bright, and close to the perceiver. However, by muting the attributes of size, distance, clarity, color, and sound of the imagery, it can ease the intensity. For example, a trauma-image that is big and bold, can be muted by making it smaller, further away, hazy, black and white, and silent. This increases emotional distance and makes it easier to tolerate. Another strategy is to imagine the image viewed through a window or on a television screen, again to increase distance. When clients are instructed to approach a scene, it is usually presented as distant and hazy. The therapist asks if they are ready to move forward. This gives clients a gentle approach and allows for the therapist to assess their reactions.

Integration after imagery reprocessing

After reprocessing, clients may need a few minutes to adjust. Then the therapist can ask how they are doing? What was it like for them? Encourage clients to pay attention to how they feel in the next few days including attention to their dreams or other thoughts that may arise. They may also wish to journal about their experiences. After reprocessing, clients should also be encouraged to take care of themselves as they integrate the experience. This may include resting, drinking water, maybe taking some quiet time, or doing something fun or nurturing for their younger self.

Chapter summary

This chapter presented an overview of the techniques for imagery reprocessing. Imagery reprocessing facilitates a constructive reorganization of the perception of trauma, which in turn modifies the associated emotional and behavioral tendencies that render people stuck in the repetitive cycling of experiential holograms. Imagery reprocessing offers a gentle path to completion and healing while engaging the visual-sensory system of the experiential mind.

Chapter 12

Integration and moving forward

This chapter shifts from an orientation about the past to an orientation towards the future. It discusses integration, what is important (e.g., values), and how to envision a desired future. It also discusses how to handle potential relapses, upsets, and triggers of past holograms including recognizing, labeling, and disengaging, as well as reprocessing booster imagery.

A case example: Delayed grief

Adam, a Caucasian male who served in the military, was recently having a flare up of PTSD issues. A few months ago, he was about to get into a fight with someone in a parking lot. Then he can't remember what happened. He went into fight/flight response and got aggressive, and then he blacked out. When he came to, he was yelling at the guy and threatening him. After that, he was really frightened because he would never want to hurt anyone.

He was also having difficulty concentrating, difficulty following through on tasks. He said part of him just gives-up, and he stops trying. He said he is easily frustrated and has difficulty thinking through a problem, like he is in a fog, unable to keep a thought. He also has been having disrupted sleep, with early morning awakening.

He was afraid to go out in public. He was having intrusive thoughts about events in the military. One incident in particular was horrific. He had blocked this memory, but then it came back in full. He said he saw a guy burned to death. He keeps thinking about the millisecond before the fire where the guy was sprayed with fuel. They were fueling an aircraft while it was running. It was a training drill. When one of the trainees disconnected the hose, the valve didn't close. The fuel sprayed like a fire hose and then it blew up in a big fire ball.

Adam was up on a ladder working out of a hanger. He was working on another plane. He was watching the guys below who were fueling a plane. He saw it happen and grabbed a fire extinguisher and slid down the ladder to spray it out. But by the time he got there it was over. He said he couldn't sleep that night. He said he never thought about it again.

DOI: 10.4324/9781003223429-14

After the incident in the parking lot, he had another memory come to him. When he was eight years old, he burned himself on a hot stove. He still has a clear memory of it. Since then, he has been thinking about the incident in the military all of the time. He has also been having a variety of emotions come to the surface. He said he has been crying and getting angry. He doesn't know why because he never did that before. He could listen to a song or think about his family and have a sudden wave of overwhelming sadness—then frustration.

Adam had social support, a good family, and he reunited with his military friends about a year ago. He has been reminiscing with them, which may also have contributed to this memory surfacing.

We discussed delayed grief and disenfranchised grief. He was open to working on regulating his nervous system. We discussed excitatory and inhibitory systems and typical reactions of PTSD. We practiced the COPE strategy—cleansing breath, observation, positive self-talk, and explanation. He said he appreciated it and that it made sense to him. He also created a positive focal point to use to distract himself and shift away from intrusive negative thoughts.

We discussed releasing the man who died that day. He was holding on to his story. Like holding on to someone else's jacket that has their name on it. He said this was helpful and appreciated talking about him and what had happened.

He said the sadness made him feel helpless. We discussed working on getting closure for the tragedies from the past. He said he liked to go to the beach where he imagined talking to people in his head. He told them that he has to let them go. He was playing with his dog, throwing a stick out in the ocean. He thought about throwing the stick as a metaphor, throwing his memories out to the ocean and letting them stay there. We discussed allowing the past deaths to go out to sea, releasing them. Imagining their souls are at peace and they are no longer his to carry. He imagined the ocean carrying them back out to sea.

We did the blue pen exercise. We used this to discuss radical acceptance. He said the exercise made a lot of sense to him. He can't change the past, it just is. We discussed how this is part of resolving grief, coming to terms with what is. In subsequent sessions he noted less tightening in his chest, less intrusive thoughts, and less anger. He said thinking about the "blue pen" has been helpful to realize it is out of his hands. He said he sees the poor man that burned that night. It's heart-breaking. He identifies with how painful that must have been.

We discussed what does he need to let him go? He said he wished he could have a ceremony at sea, a formal ceremony, with a chaplain saying a few words. We discussed thinking of doing a virtual or symbolic ceremony. He said that would be nice and he would come up with something to symbolize him and then release him with honor and respect.

Integration and moving forward

Adam had delayed grief that surfaced abruptly—maybe because he stopped working, or maybe because he was meeting with old friends from the military. He had intrusive thoughts that brought him back to his time in the military. Once these thoughts were activated, associated memories also came to the surface (e.g., burning himself on a stove, and deaths of family members). It was intruding on his thoughts, mood, sleep, and cognitive function. We worked on affect regulation skills and then acceptance. Adam witnessed an event and was stuck in complicated grief, but he did not personalize the incident or blame himself. He did mention that he had some self-blame at the time, he thought maybe he should have gotten there sooner to help, but let that go because he knew that he really couldn't. He understood it was a thought related to his feeling of being helpless. Instead, his task was coming to acceptance, and releasing his grief for this young man.

Instead of imagery reprocessing, he opted for a symbolic release. Imagery reprocessing is convenient as it can be done in a therapist's office. However, a symbolic gesture, ritual, or ceremony can be equally as powerful. These efforts also reach the experiential system as they are experiential in nature. They can also be shared with others intensifying the experience. In *Warrior Renew* (2014), the final community exercise is a virtual releasing ceremony where each person releases something into a virtual fire pit, and the community affirms. It is symbolic of letting go of one's hologram and experiencing a physical and emotional liberation.

What happens after reprocessing?

Once people feel complete with their past, they may come in with another issue or concern for the future. This is a positive sign, as instead of focusing on the past (e.g., focusing on the rear-view mirror), they are now looking through the windshield, at the road ahead. Once free of the past or anything that has been holding them back, it begs to ask, what is next, how does one move forward? For many, their holograms have been a significant pervasive part of their life for many years. For some, releasing the past may be a new crisis, disorienting, and yet full of possibilities. Clients are asked to consider, how do they want to move forward in their lives, what is important, and what outcomes would they like to create? They may explore values, goals, and take some time to be calm, to listen to their heart or inner awareness. For some, this may be foreign and uncomfortable to really consider what they want. Clients are encouraged to dream and imagine. What moves their heart forward? Similar to the focusing exercises, they can sit quietly and ask themselves what do they really want? Utilizing similar skills used in reprocessing, clients are invited to envision their future.

Writing a letter to one's future self

Instead of rescripting the past, clients can script their future. Where would they like to be in several years and what would they like to say to their future self? This could include writing a letter to one's future self— what might one's future self look like, or be doing? Then they can imagine meeting their future self and having a conversation. This is creating a hologram to some extent, a future hologram.

If you could meet your *future self*, what would you say and what would you like your future self to say back?

Imagery message to one's future self

"Up ahead you see a grassy clearing. There is a big boulder resting on the bank of a stream. You walk up to the boulder and see that it is smooth and shaped in such a way that it would be very comfortable to lean against. Imagine sitting by the stream with your back resting on the rock. You look into the stream and it appears so clean and refreshing. Look around and find a leaf. Hold the leaf in your hands and think of a message to send to your future self. Now blow your message into the leaf so that it is fused into its fibers. When you are ready, and only when you are ready, toss the leaf with your message into the stream. Watch as the stream carries the leaf away. Know that your message has been sent. Take in a deep breath. Are you complete with this scene?"

Post-treatment plan

After reprocessing, clients may feel motivated to move forward on goals and are ready to commit to living consistent with their values. Nonetheless, there will be tests along the way, such as reminders, anniversaries, trauma triggers, or something in the present that initiates an automatic memory of the past releasing a cascade of neurochemicals. Even if someone knows they are lovable, worthy, good enough, or safe, likely there will be something to challenge these new beliefs. This is why having a good post-treatment plan is helpful. This may include a plan for on-going practice of emotion regulation skills.

Follow-up care

The current-age self is now the caretaker of one's past self. With awareness comes responsibility. Enacting behaviors that replicate old patterns is hurtful and disrespectful to one's younger and current self. Clients may need follow-up support and skills to address deficits.

If someone had a neglect hologram, knowing the impact of neglect, it is no longer okay to neglect oneself and one's needs. This may lead to needing skills for boundary setting, communication skills, and how to consider one's own needs as well as everyone else's.

If someone had a rejection hologram, then they are at risk for self-criticism and rejecting or judging oneself and others. This may lead to needing skills in self-acceptance, loving kindness, and continued affect regulation practices.

If someone had a betrayal hologram, they may be at risk for over- or under-trusting others. They may need to learn skills in discernment, incremental trust, communication skills, and continued affect regulation practices.

If someone had an endangerment hologram, they may have trauma triggers, experience bouts of fear, and have difficulty trusting. They may need skills in discernment, boundaries, communication, self-acceptance, loving kindness, and affect regulation practices.

If someone experienced complicated grief, a traumatic event, or moral injury they may encounter something that reminds them of their past. It will bring up old feelings that will peak and subside. The upset will be temporary, possibly intense, or maybe not as intense as it would have been in the past. The experience can be felt and observed at the same time, like watching clothes in a washing machine—staying grounded and not getting caught up in it. It will pass and fade back to the past where it belongs.

Addressing temporary relapses of old patterns

It is normal and expected that something or someone will activate an old feeling related to one's hologram. These are deeply ingrained and may automatically arise. Most people will be challenged with reminders or triggers. If or when something triggers an old feeling or old pattern, it can be upsetting but does not have to mean more than what it is, a reminder of something from the past. The challenge is to recognize it for what it is. "This is my hologram." It is familiar, but it is also an illusion. It is not true. It is based on a feeling and a belief. It helps to label it. As one client said every time, she felt judgmental, she would catch herself and say, "Oh that's my hologram." It is recognizable, and something to keep in check. Then she can intentionally disengage from negative thinking and practice self-compassion.

Strategies to address a momentary relapse include: label what is, "that's my hologram," engage emotion regulation, provide comfort to oneself, engage in positive self-talk, remember the feeling will pass, and engage in a positive image or thought (e.g., a positive focal point). This is a counter-image that will help soothe and disengage from the negative thinking.

How to disengage from negative thinking

Don't entertain the guest, but rather escort the thought right out of the house. Negative thinking is an unpleasant guest who will take over your mind if you let it. Just kindly say, "No thank you. Not today." And refocus on something else, perhaps a positive focal point, or anything that helps shift your attention. Or simply do a big cleansing breath, inhale through the nose, and out with a sigh, letting it all go. Do something that will make you feel better (e.g., a walk, watch a comedy, listen to music, talk to a friend, etc.).

Booster reprocessing

Some may find that a booster imagery reprocessing session is helpful. One's current-age self can go back and visit one's younger self, offering reassurance, giving a hug, letting them know they are loved and are brave, that they are doing a great job, and one's current-age self is still here to provide safety, comfort, and love. Similar to imagery reprocessing, start with being grounded, relaxed, and safe. Imagine walking along a country road to engage the imagery, activating the senses. Then approach the place of the younger self. Anchored as one's current age, imagine seeing the younger self, moving towards the self, connecting, and offering a healing communication. The therapist offers, "Is there anything you want to say? Is there anything you want to do?" In a booster session, the client may want to leave a gift, or symbol as a reminder of something positive for the younger self. For example, leaving a butterfly, and every time the current self sees a butterfly, it will be a pleasant reminder of the connection with one's younger self.

Traumatic growth

Post-traumatic growth is a concept developed by psychologists Richard Tedeschi, Ph.D., and Lawrence Calhoun, Ph.D. It is the idea that after going through a significant event, it can have profound effects including some positive ones, such as a new outlook on life or motivating meaningful changes. The *Posttraumatic Growth Inventory* (Tedeschi & Calhoun, 1996) examines five areas for growth: appreciation of life, relationships with others, new possibilities in life, personal strength, and spiritual change.

This may manifest as increased gratitude and reverence for life. It may mean valuing positive relationships, holding boundaries with unsupportive relationships, or seeking new relationships. It could mean stepping back and re-evaluating one's values and reflecting upon what is most important. It could lead to an increased openness to experiences or motivation to engage in activities that one has always wanted to do. It may lead to increased self-esteem, self-care, and attending to one's needs. Growth can be choosing to live free of one's hologram, being intentional, and becoming more aware of oneself and others.

It is a powerful realization, that the past does not need to define or limit one's future moving forward. It is a step towards self-determination, and living life with intentionality, and liberty.

It is acknowledged that not everyone will be welcoming of this concept, and it is in no way meant to minimize the horror of going through trauma, abuse, or maltreatment. These are painful and life-altering experiences. However, it is worth considering as a result of going through such challenging and intense experiences, is there something meaningful that can be gained? Even with substantial losses, there may be something that shifts as a result—maybe a new respect or appreciation for good things in life, perhaps motivation to make a difference or help others? It is ironic, but for some, their worst experience may bring forward a great opportunity.

Aghajani et al. (2021) conducted a study aimed to determine the effects of holographic reprocessing therapy on cognitive flexibility and posttraumatic growth in women with breast cancer who underwent mastectomy. Those who had holographic reprocessing along with chemotherapy had significantly improved cognitive flexibility and traumatic growth compared to those who received chemotherapy alone. Building upon the work of Mehrparvar et al. (2017), who also found holographic reprocessing helped women with cancer, the authors recommended holographic reprocessing therapy as a complementary treatment without adverse effects along with medical treatments for breast cancer patients. In these studies, holographic reprocessing helped women shift to a positive attitude when facing a serious life-threatening disease. This is a particularly powerful finding, suggesting that the treatment is not only effective in reducing negative symptoms (e.g., depression, anxiety, negative thoughts) as found in several randomized clinical trials (Katz et al., 2014b; Basharpoor et al., 2011), but also supports a factor of growth.

One factor that may contribute to growth could be improved cognitive flexibility. Holographic reprocessing utilizes several strategies to help people see multiple truths, from an observer vantage point, or from the perspective of others involved in a trauma. It asks clients to consider new ways to understand or make sense of their experience without refuting their original perceptions. This process is pivotal for many who engage in this treatment. Evidence supporting effectiveness of this process has been collected by Salehi and colleagues (Salehi et al., 2019; Salehi et al., 2020; Salehi & Beshlideh, 2020), who examined the outcomes of applying holographic reprocessing with clients with depression and a recent suicide attempt. Their research found those who engaged in holographic reprocessing had significantly improved cognitive flexibility, and improved social adjustment (Salehi et al., 2019; Salehi et al., 2020; Salehi & Beshlideh, 2020).

Post-treatment engagement

An important phase of healing is what happens after a trauma-focused therapy. This may include follow-up therapeutic groups, or classes, but more importantly, what attitude will the client embrace? Where will they place their focus? This may lead to a discussion about creating a future-oriented positive focal point; perhaps thinking about goals, desired experiences, or a new self-image. Some like to place words or images as reminders and as a way to stay motivated. After imagery reprocessing, some may want to engage in something meaningful or to make a contribution to others. This is discussed as pro-social engagement which can have many positive health effects including activation (getting up and out of the house), improved socializing, improved self-esteem, and overall positive feelings. Although research shows inconsistent findings about direct effects on emotions, some feel strongly that practicing gratitude or performing kindness activities improves a sense of happiness, as was found in the study of Rowland and Curry (2019).

Saying "Yes" and saying "No"

Engaging in activities may be a big step for some, especially for those who have spent many years avoiding people and activities. It may be helpful to discuss embracing an appropriate yes-attitude towards new experiences and opportunities. As discussed in *Psychology Today* blog (Katz, 2021), "the word yes by definition, is a positive affirmation, and a word of agreement. It opens dialogue, allows for possibilities, encourages further inquiry, and moves people forward."

However, embracing yes may not be easy after experiencing trauma. What may have started as protection can develop into a pattern of avoidance. Saying no is an efficient barrier and stops whatever is being requested, offered, or asked and essentially brings a conversation to a halt (Katz, 2021). It is a simple and elegant way to avoid new or potentially threatening experiences.

However, is avoiding the situation truly avoiding something negative, or is it allowing fear to dictate one's life choices? Is declining an invitation or not engaging in an activity, based on a fear that something bad could potentially happen, but not necessarily likely to happen? Simply imagining a possible negative or dangerous outcome does not mean that it will likely occur. This is *what-if* thinking, such as "What if something terrible happens?" That thought alone will trigger the fight/flight/freeze response as if it was actually happening (even though it is not), and can derail one's plans. Avoiding new experiences because of fear keeps people stuck recycling old feelings from the past. Instead, *what-is* thinking will help people stay grounded in this moment (e.g., what is happening right now). *What-is* thinking coupled with slow deep breathing will help calm one's nervous system. Calming is the first step to assessing realistic levels of threat or danger.

Once calm and ready to determine if one wants to engage in an activity or not, it is important to consider one's own needs as well as others to be able to authentically answer either yes or no. It can be helpful to practice focusing skills to detect, "*What am I feeling?*" "*Is this fear? Or is this wisdom?*" This is an important skill to acquire. In the meantime, a quick tool can be used to help decide, the five magic words when someone makes a request: "Let me think about it" (Katz, 2014). This gives people time to think, "*What do I want to do? Do I want to go to this event? Do I want to help this person?*" It is helpful to remember to honor one's time, feelings, resources, and finances. What are the goals, values, and life-choices that they want to move towards? Once clear about one's goals, and out of the grips of guilt and obligation, the person can decide if they want to go, or help, or not. This frees oneself to be able to genuinely say yes or no. Sometimes no is the healthiest response as it upholds boundaries, and honors one's commitments and integrity. The goal is to be able to authentically say yes or no and mean it.

In the 2008 movie, *Yes Man* (Soller et al., 2008), the main character played by Jim Carrey transforms his life by saying "Yes" to every request and opportunity. Of course, this was played to the extreme for comedy. But the idea is to welcome life experiences. "(Yes) fosters collaboration, and problem solving. It is a catalyst for growth and change. Ideas are nurtured to the sound of yes. Possibilities emerge, new pathways are forged, and… yes, change does happen" (Katz, 2021).

Ask your client if they are willing to give up the life they have, for the life they want.

Are they willing to do something different?

Sometimes happiness comes in different packages than what is expected. It's not about controlling but rather seeing opportunities, being open to change, and allowing life to unfold. After reprocessing, the question is, what would your client like to create in their life? What would bring joy, good health, and supportive relationships? What could they say "yes" to that moves their body forward? Icek Ajzen, Ph.D. (1991) developed the theory of planned behavior and found that setting an intention significantly increases the likelihood that one will do the behavior. In other words, thinking about an action occurs before someone engages in the action. In this case, thinking about what is desired in life is going to help generate ideas, set goals, and make plans to engage in these behaviors.

Tips for moving towards a desired life:

1 Define your values (what's most important to you?), dreams, desires; what do you want? If you had time, money, ability, what would you want to do? Even if initially, this seems unrealistic, what is the essence that you want and how can you move towards a version that is realistic?

2 What are your goals? Outcome goals are great for motivation and for looking for opportunities, followed by process goals, or specific steps to get there

3 It can be helpful to design a visual reminder of what one wants in their life. This helps people stay focused and to motivate them to move towards their desired direction, sometimes in spite of fear or negative thoughts

Opportunities are numerous, but it takes being open to see them and welcome them into your life. Being able to say "no" is important when holding one's boundaries and asserting your own needs. And being able to say "yes" is equally important to welcome new experiences into one's life.

With each new breath, we inhale opening to life,
and with each exhale, we release all that no longer serves.

Chapter summary

This chapter presented strategies for integration and moving forward. This includes imagining sending a message to one's future self either through imagery or writing a letter. It also suggests strategies for post-treatment follow-up to include a plan for relapse of old patterns and addressing other issues for continued improvement. It also suggests considering positive aspects gained as a result of one's past experience framed as traumatic growth. Finally, it discussed strategies for moving forward towards a desired life.

Part 3

Status in the field

Chapter 13

Comparison to other trauma therapies

This chapter starts with an example of imagery reprocessing. The body of the chapter presents a discussion comparing holographic reprocessing to other trauma treatments and to other imagery-based treatments. It discusses the strengths and limitations of each and the unique features of holographic reprocessing therapy.

Case example of imagery reprocessing

In this example, the client, Tom, had a neglect interpersonal experiential hologram. He felt unresolved from his past when his father left him (and his mother) when he was a child. He said he rarely had interactions with his father. We had discussed that it is important to understand that his father's decision to move was not based on his love or lack of love for his son.

THERAPIST: Tom, when I listen to the issues you discuss in therapy with me, it all seems to stem from your feelings that your father doesn't like or love you.

CLIENT: Yes, I do feel that way; I have felt that way ever since I was a little boy. Rationally, I know otherwise, but I still feel that my dad moved away because he didn't love me.

THERAPIST: Tom, the fact that your father moved away when you were young seems to have had a pretty strong impact on you. I'm wondering if you would be comfortable doing an exercise in which we visited your younger self.

CLIENT: Okay, I can try that.

THERAPIST: Okay, you are you at your current age right now... and your younger self is how old?

CLIENT: He's 7.

THERAPIST: We are going to do a guided imagery for relaxation and then imagine meeting your younger self. I know we've talked about this before, but do you have an idea of what you would like to say to your younger self? and what you would like to do?

DOI: 10.4324/9781003223429-16

CLIENT: Yes, I do.

THERAPIST: Okay, settle into your chair, feet on the ground… feeling your body supported by the chair. Let's do a signal breath, deep breath in through the nose… hold it at the top… and exhale through the mouth. Signaling to the body it's time to relax. And breathe… a little slower and a little deeper. Releasing your shoulders on the next exhale. Feeling your whole body sinking into the chair. Continue breathing.…

Okay, imagine that you are taking a relaxing walk through the forest. You are walking along a path, enjoying the nature around you, beautiful trees, blue sky… take in a deep breath, smelling fresh air. You continue walking down the path, and in the far distance you see a house. As you get closer, you realize that the house is the one that you lived in as a kid. The house is far away so you cannot see it clearly. As you continue to walk towards the house, you can see the house much clearer. On a scale of 1 to 10 with 1 being very relaxed and 10 being extremely tense, where are you now Tom?

CLIENT: I am about a 3.

THERAPIST: Good. And continue to breathe. You are you as your current age self, feet grounded, standing before the door to your childhood home. (*Pause*) When you are ready, open the door to the house.

CLIENT: (*Takes a deep breath*) Okay.

THERAPIST: When you are ready step inside the house… and what do you see?

CLIENT: Okay…I see a little boy sitting on the floor playing with some toys. His mother is in the kitchen cooking, and his grandmother is sitting on the couch. The little boy's older brother is outside playing.

THERAPIST: What is the little boy feeling.

CLIENT: He feels sad and lonely. He wonders why his dad has moved away.

THERAPIST: Now you, as a man in his mid-20s, what would you like to say to the little boy who is feeling sad and lonely about his dad who moved away?

CLIENT: I would sit next to him on the floor and put my arm around him and tell him he's a great kid.

THERAPIST: Go ahead.

CLIENT: (*Using an extremely soft voice*) You are a great kid and everything will be alright.

THERAPIST: Anything else?

CLIENT: (*Continues to use a very soft voice*) Your father did not move because he did not love you. He and your mother were having problems and he knew he could make a better life for himself.

THERAPIST: Anything else you would like to say to him Tom?

CLIENT: I'm always going to be here for you. I'm going to take care of you and comfort you.

THERAPIST: (*Pause*)… anything else?

CLIENT: No. The little boy is happy that I came to visit him today. He knows... that he's loved.

THERAPIST: Ok Tom, then let's go back on the country road... looking at the trees, blue sky above. Find yourself back in this chair, feet on the ground. Inhaling through the nose, and out with a sigh. Stretching your arms and yawning...

CLIENT: That was amazing. I feel really good. It was weird to see myself as a little boy. Wow.

Holographic reprocessing: A unique approach

Holographic reprocessing, as stated, draws upon CET and integrates aspects of various treatment components organized into a coherent model. There are parallel aspects to treatments such as schema therapy (Young, 1999) where themes of re-enactments are identified. Similar to cognitive therapy (Ehlers & Clark, 2000), perceptions are shifted utilizing cognitive-based techniques relying on the rational mind to reappraise emotional-based thinking. Holographic reprocessing uses similar experiential therapy techniques (Gendlin,1996) such as being aware of physical sensations and paying attention to the body "moving forward" when there is an experiential connection. It uses similar aspects of narrative therapy (White, 2007) such as being the observer and author of one's life; and similar elements from acceptance and commitment therapy (ACT: Hayes et al., 1999), such as using metaphors to communicate concepts and encouraging clients to be future-oriented in a self-determined way consistent with one's values.

However, when compared to treatments for trauma, holographic reprocessing is distinct in many ways. Holographic reprocessing uses the model of a hologram. Wrapped within its language is the concept that perceptions feel real but are not necessarily true. They are part true but not the whole truth. Similarly, shifting perceptions is facilitated through a holistic reappraisal considering context from the observer vantage point. This technique utilizes the skills of mentalization to consider perceptions outside of oneself such as considering the agendas, perceptions, and feelings of others. This is in contrast from the cognitive-behavioral approach of arguing for and against a specific thought with the focus solely on the client. These thoughts are labeled as problematic thinking; whereas in holographic reprocessing, this type of thinking is considered a natural product of emotional thinking. Holographic reprocessing uses novel metaphors and strategies throughout.

The most popular evidence-based trauma treatments are prolonged exposure (PE) (Foa et al., 2007), cognitive processing therapy (CPT) (Resick & Schnicke, 1996), and eye movement desensitization and reprocessing (EMDR: Shapiro, 2001). Many studies support their efficacy. Lewis et al. (2020) reviewed 114 randomized clinical trials of treatments for PTSD and found that the strongest supporting evidence was for trauma-focused cognitive behavioral treatments PE and CPT, and EMDR.

Prolonged exposure (PE)

PE therapy has been one of the most widely practiced and researched treatments for PTSD. PE consists of 12 sessions addressing symptoms associated with PTSD based on the theory that people will try to ward-off intrusive thoughts and avoid trauma-reminders, even when those reminders are not inherently dangerous. In other words, if someone was attacked by someone wearing a red jacket, smoking a cigar, in a park, then anything associated with the attack might evoke symptoms of danger and fear. The person may then avoid anything that could trigger this reaction, even neutral objects, such as red jackets, cigars, and parks. Using imaginal and in vivo exposure, clients reduce their fear, desensitize to memories, and learn that they can venture to places that they were avoiding. The treatment also involves retelling the event of trauma from beginning to end as vividly as possible and then clients are instructed to listen to the recording multiple times daily. The event is retold again in session and aspects that may be particularly emotional are labeled as hot spots. More time is spent retelling details of these points of the narrative. Conversational processing can occur after the retelling.

Shortcomings of exposure therapy

While those who benefit from PE have marked improvements in symptoms, it is not beneficial for everyone. One issue is high dropout rates, especially in naturalistic trials (see Najavits, 2015), possibly due to perceived discomfort associated with the treatment. Research has attempted to identify who may or may not benefit from this treatment with mixed results. Anxiety and hyperarousal may potentially be one factor predicting poorer outcomes. van Minnen and Hagenaars (2002) found in a sample of 45 participants with mixed trauma 21 improved, 13 did not, and 11 dropped out of PE treatment. Those who did not improve had higher anxiety at the onset. Those who did improve had higher rates of habituation after the first session. This is supported by a neuroimaging study where McCurry et al. (2020) found that hyperarousal was a factor that diminished neural habituation to aversive stimuli in a sample of combat-exposed veterans.

Another component is that PE is narrow in its focus. Ehlers and colleagues (2005) found that individuals whose memories during the reliving of the trauma reflected mental defeat or the absence of mental planning showed little improvement with exposure. They also found that individuals with an overall feeling of alienation or permanent change following the trauma also had poor response with exposure. They conclude that these clients may require cognitive restructuring in addition to the exposure. For some, activating trauma-related emotions will only yield benefit if there is some recasting or restructuring of the emotional memory (Littrell, 1998).

One possible explanation as to why exposure therapy has produced positive results is that there might be some spontaneous restructuring of the emotional memory by the mere act of exposure. In PE, clients are instructed to retell their memory of trauma as if they are experiencing it. However, after the client recants the events multiple times, 20, 30, 70 times, they seem to have a spontaneous shift. PE theory would say it is due to habituation.

However, holographic reprocessing offers another explanation. Repeated exposure of retelling one's story shifts the focus from the field (as if re-experiencing the memory) to the observer vantage point (as if viewing from afar). From this perspective, the shift occurs when a client hears themselves telling the story. It becomes a story. The client no longer experiences the associated symptoms as if reliving the experience. From the observer vantage point, they may spontaneously gain perspective, have insights, or shift blame. In holographic reprocessing, the detailed retelling of the story part is skipped, and clients are systematically led through strategies to gain perspective utilizing the observer vantage point.

Comparing and contrasting holographic reprocessing and PE

Both PE and holographic reprocessing require: 1) focus on an unresolved issue, and 2) a corrective emotional experience (see Alexander & French, 1946). For PE, the target focus is of the *fear structure* or the associated fears with an event of trauma. For holographic reprocessing, the focus is on the *experiential hologram* or the negative perception of self in relation to others and/or the world. Both structures are learned associations developed from trauma. The ensuing corrective emotional experience counters the learning from the trauma. In other words, both treatments emphasize feeling differently (e.g., PE: the goal in vivo exposure is to feel relaxed and safe, and for holographic reprocessing the goal could be to feel safe, loved, forgiven, and/or accepted). Both treatments also utilize imagery as a way to connect with the experiential system and conversational processing to consolidate the experiential learning within the rational or cognitive system.

Nonetheless, these treatments approach learning from recall of trauma in opposite ways. In PE, recall is from the field vantage point, while in holographic reprocessing, recall is from the observer vantage point. In PE, the use of the field vantage point activates affective and physiological activation. On the other hand, the observer vantage point minimizes affective sensations, and instead, facilitates a distanced view that enhances a broader perspective of a scene or event. This is consistent with the McIsaac and Eich studies (2002, 2004) where recall of memories from the field vantage point was associated with affective and physiological states (e.g., "I felt nervous"),

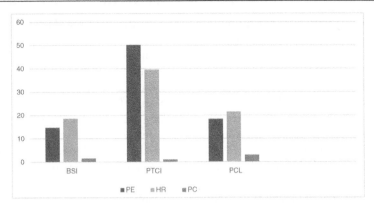

PE= Prolonged exposure, HR= Holographic reprocessing, PC= Present-centered, BSI-
18= Brief symptom inventory, PTCI= Posttraumatic cognitions inventory, PCL= PTSD
Checklist IV

Figure 13.1 Mean change scores of symptoms after treatment for women veterans
who experienced military sexual trauma (Katz et al., 2014b).
PE = prolonged exposure, HR = holographic reprocessing, PC = present-centered, BSI-
18 = brief symptom inventory, PTCI = posttraumatic cognitions inventory, PCL= PTSD
Checklist IV.

while recall of memories from the observer vantage point was associated
with recall of spatial relationships between objects and people in the scene
(e.g., "I saw myself sitting next to the ball"). In PE, recall from the field
vantage point helps with desensitization. In holographic reprocessing, the
observer vantage point helps clients gain perspective and form new meanings
about their experience.

A randomized clinical trial compared PE to holographic reprocessing and
a present centered (PC) control group (Katz et al., 2014b). Fifty-one female
veterans with a history of sexual trauma were randomly assigned to one of
three conditions: PE, holographic reprocessing, and PC (17 in each group).
Holographic reprocessing and PE treatments both led to greater decreases in
symptoms of anxiety, depression, and PTSD compared to the PC control
group but did not differ from each other. Holographic reprocessing produced a
significantly lower dropout rate 1/17 (6%) compared to PE 7/17 (41%) and PC
6/17 (35%).

Cognitive processing therapy

CPT is a 12-session manualized therapy for PTSD which teaches clients to
challenge and modify unhelpful, irrational, and incorrect thoughts and
beliefs about oneself and others related to a traumatic experience (Resick

et. al., 2016). There are five themes addressed in the treatment: safety, trust, power and control, esteem, and intimacy. CPT uses Socratic questions to help clients more accurately appraise their cognitive stuck points and progress toward recovery. Clients learn to complete thought records which helps them confront their beliefs and automatic thinking. Completing weekly thought records gives clients a framework to articulate their thoughts and evaluate supporting evidence. CPT focuses on a single target event. It may begin with having clients write a narrative of their trauma account or an impact statement. These are used to identify negative or limiting thinking, and types of problematic thinking, for example, jumping to conclusions, overgeneralization, catastrophizing, and emotional reasoning.

Holographic reprocessing and CPT share similar therapeutic goals to shift perceptions about the attributions and assumptions made about the self and others. Both target changing or modifying cognitions. For CPT the focus is on modifying specific thoughts and beliefs. For holographic reprocessing the focus is on considering context for understanding the experience in a new way.

Shortcomings of cognitive processing therapy

CPT is well-established as an evidence-based treatment and is highly recommended for treating negative or limited thinking as a result of experiencing a trauma. However, CPT is not well-suited for everyone. It is heavily reliant on completing homework which may not appeal to some clients especially if they struggle with completing assignments. It also targets a specific event of trauma. If clients have multiple traumas, they typically pick one event as their target event. This may be difficult for those who have trauma across the life-span and with multiple co-morbidities in addition to PTSD. CPT is also not well-suited for group therapy. A study found that individual CPT treatment produced stronger results in reducing PTSD in a military population than group treatment (Resick et al., 2017). However, even those who received individual CPT therapy, 50% still had significant symptoms.

Another potential short-falling of this approach is that clients may state that they know an event (e.g., trauma) was not their fault; however, at a deep emotional level, they may continue to feel guilty or ashamed. Using logic or collecting rational evidence alone may not be enough to reach clients at these deeper levels. Furthermore, traumatic memories seem to lack a verbal narrative as traumatic experiences are encoded in the experiential system at the somatosensory level in the form of physical sensations and visual images (van der Kolk, 1994; van der Kolk et al., 1997). Because there has been a halting of the processing of these experiences, they remain at the experiential level without the abstraction of a narrative context.

Comparing and contrasting holographic reprocessing and CPT

In contrast to CPT, holographic reprocessing takes a holistic approach in which the goal is to reprocess patterns of emotional and behavioral tendencies. It also does not focus on specific automatic thoughts. Problematic thinking is conceptualized as a by-product of emotional thinking of the experiential mind. Holographic reprocessing uses a blend of cognitive and experiential techniques to help clients shift perceptions at a deep experiential level. While holographic reprocessing uses a rational-based discussion, the focus is on considering context and new meanings. It helps clients see multiple truths to assist with cognitive reframing (e.g., understanding something from a new point of view) in conjunction with experiential-based procedures such as imagery reprocessing.

In the cognitive model, limiting perceptions are discredited as maladaptive or distorted, whereas in holographic reprocessing negative personalized beliefs are understood as making sense given the context and point of view of the person experiencing the event. Holographic reprocessing does not refute a person's perceptions but rather holds a context for emotional thinking and states that there are multiple points of view. Holographic reprocessing encourages clients to view all the characters in a scene including oneself, as well as environmental factors, to assist seeing a broader context for the event. This facilitates an objective reappraisal or understanding of the whole scene, by considering factors outside of oneself.

A randomized clinical trial compared CPT to holographic reprocessing and a present-centered control group (Basharpoor et al., 2011; Narimani et al., 2011; Narimani et al., 2013). Out of 10,000 male high-school students, 1,000 were randomly screened and 129 were identified as having experienced a trauma. Sixty of them were randomly assigned to either holographic reprocessing, CPT, or a control group (20 in each group). Both active treatments had greater decreases in posttraumatic cognitions, and symptoms of anxiety, depression, and PTSD compared to the control group. Holographic reprocessing was superior to CPT in reducing anxiety, dissociation, and PTSD symptoms, while CPT was superior in reducing depression (Basharpoor et al., 2011, Narimani et al., 2011; Narimani et al., 2013). Holographic reprocessing also produced stronger results than CPT on the subscale of *self-blame,* and with a dropout of 10% compared to CPT with 20%.

Eye movement desensitization and reprocessing therapy

EMDR is a structured therapy that encourages clients to focus on the worst parts of a trauma memory while simultaneously experiencing bilateral stimulation (typically horizontal eye movements), which is associated with a reduction in the vividness and emotion associated with trauma memories. EMDR therapy does not require talking in detail about the distressing issue or completing homework assignments between sessions. EMDR uses imagery exposure coupled with eye movements which helps make the process more tolerable. EMDR helps to connect thoughts and images to body sensations and tensions. Some people report significant improvement within a few sessions, while others may need to be in treatment longer. The type of problem, life circumstances, and trauma history determine how many EMDR sessions are necessary. A brief version, called Flash, expedites the process to reduce negative sensations associated with a specific trauma, and can be achieved in 1–2 sessions. For example, Flash can reduce anxiety and body tension related to a discrete event such as a motor vehicle accident. EMDR assists with reduction of trauma related anxiety, PTSD, and avoided emotional processing. It is presented as a desensitization procedure, while holographic reprocessing is not about desensitization.

Comparing holographic reprocessing and trauma treatments

Ultimately, all of these trauma treatments, PE, CPT, EMDR, and holographic reprocessing, lead to disengaging negative affect from memories and thought patterns. While PE, CPT, and EMDR have a solid evidence base, they are not effective for everyone or for all traumas. PE, CPT, and EMDR tend to have a narrow scope by focusing on a particular event of trauma, and they offer limited training in acquiring new coping skills, addressing meaning, or enhancing positive emotional factors as their target for the intervention. PE and CPT can be emotionally demanding both in session and between sessions due to requirements of homework and focus on details of trauma events.

Several studies have reported high dropout rates particularly for PE in pragmatic trials in real world conditions (e.g., 68% in Garcia et al., 2011; 79% in DeViva, 2014; and 72% in Zayfert et al., 2005). Najavits (2015) discusses the importance of evaluating the efficacy of a treatment not only based on measurable outcomes but also on its ability to retain participants under real-world conditions. This is particularly significant as Hoge et al. (2014) stated, "Dropping out of care is clearly the most important predictor of treatment failure; therefore, the most promising strategies to improve efficacy of evidence-based treatments will be those that address engagement, therapeutic rapport, and retention" (p.1002).

In contrast, holographic reprocessing has a notably low dropout rate with several pragmatic trials in real world conditions. Although this is based on relatively few studies compared to the other treatments, the results are promising. For example, Katz et al. (2008) found holographic reprocessing was associated with significant decreases on posttraumatic cognitions with zero dropout in a sample of women veterans who experienced sexual trauma.

Holographic reprocessing, unlike the other treatments, works to build emotional regulation skills, and positive factors such as improved secure attachment, self-esteem, cognitive flexibility, and optimism. PTSD may be associated with a host of cognitive-emotional deficits not specifically addressed in other trauma treatments. For example, Daneshvar et al. (2022) found those who had PTSD had significantly lower scores on cognitive flexibility, self-compassion including self-kindness, common humanity, and mindfulness and significantly higher scores of self-judgment, isolation, and over-identification. Thus, addressing these factors, as holographic reprocessing does, may be an important contribution to treating PTSD.

Table 13.1 A comparison of trauma treatments

TOPIC	Holographic reprocessing	PE	CPT	EMDR
Vantage point for memory recall	Observer/ distanced	Field/ immersed until habituation	Field/ immersed then utilizing the logical observer	Field/ immersed then bilateral stimulation
Level of arousal	Low	High to moderate to low	Moderate to low	Low
Content focus	Examine patterns and context; seek why someone has symptoms	Recalling what happened as if experiencing it, exposure to feared places	Examining thoughts/ beliefs related to topics, confront emotional stuck points	Images of trauma, associations, memories, while focusing on bilateral stimuli
Mechanism of change	Reappraisal by considering context, expanding one's perspective, then offering compassion via imagery to one's younger self	With repeated exposure, fear is desensitized. Habituation to fear. Working through hot spots of emotional content with more exposure	Confronting emotional thinking using thought records, evaluating evidence for and against target thoughts	Revisiting images while staying calm through bilateral stimulation
Amount of homework	Low: Practice skills, write a letter to one's younger self	High: Daily repeated exposure, in vivo exposure	High: Daily completion of thought records	None
Skills acquired	Many skills for affect regulation, and acceptance, many metaphors to gain perspective, skills for imagery rescripting	Breathing retraining, tolerance	Thought records to confront emotional thinking	Not focused on acquiring skills

Holographic reprocessing also has limitations and is not meant for everyone. Those who want to focus on the retelling of their trauma, or want to address desensitization would be better served by the other treatments (Table 13.1). It is also not for those who have difficulty considering different points of view, or difficulty engaging in imagery. It has been successfully implemented with clients who had trauma and substance use disorders (in a residential substance abuse treatment center) and with clients who have had a suicide attempt within the past year. However, it is not recommended for anyone in a current crisis, who is actively abusing alcohol or drugs, or having active or very recent suicidal (or homicidal) ideation. It is also not recommended for those who are highly dissociative who would need focused work on affect regulation.

Comparing holographic reprocessing to imagery-based therapies

Several treatments utilize imagery to evoke a corrective emotional experience, including imagery similar to holographic reprocessing's visiting one's younger self. Examples of these treatments are schema therapy's limited reparenting (Young et al., 2003), security priming Gillath and Karantzas (2019), imagery rescripting (Holmes et al., 2007), and adaptive disclosure (AD: Litz et al., 2016).

Schema therapy and limited reparenting

Schema therapy and limited reparenting (Young et al., 2003) is based on attachment theory. The therapist helps clients meet their early childhood unmet needs, or maladaptive schemas, by fostering a secure attachment with the therapist. Early maladaptive schemas are self-defeating emotional and cognitive patterns established from childhood and repeat throughout life. The therapist delivers appropriate nurturance, firmness, self-disclosure, confrontation, playfulness, and setting of limits to meet core needs of a client and, thereby, improve the maladaptive schemas. Limited reparenting involves welcoming and encouraging therapist dependency. Through resonance with the therapist, the therapist models and teaches the client to regulate affect which becomes internalized by the client to develop healthy adult behavior and ultimately, autonomy.

Strategies used in limited reparenting involves reaching parts or modes of the client such as the vulnerable child, or angry child. The therapist offers reassurance, being firm with or setting limits, or provides constructive outlets. In addition, it often requires that the therapist help the patient fight punitive, demanding, or subjugating parent modes or schemas. These steps can be facilitated with guided imagery and imagery rescripting. The client recalls painful memories and imagines revising the imagery in order to get their needs met. The therapist may enter the image serving as a healthy parent. Clients may also express anger towards those who hurt them in the imagery role-play. Imagery from grief or trauma is used as a way to rework memories and imagine an outcome that promotes safety and protection.

Security priming

Security primes activate a sense of attachment security by making mental representations in one's memory more accessible and salient. Gillath and Karantzas (2019) reviewed 20 published studies to determine the effects of security priming. They found security priming, especially via guided imagery or visualization, was associated with beneficial effects across a diverse set of domains. The effects were especially strong among anxiously attached individuals leading to long-term alterations. Therefore, it is possible to effect enduring changes to people's attachment styles through repeated security priming practiced over time (Carnelley & Rowe, 2007, Gillath et al., 2008). These state-level changes that are practiced and maintained for long periods of time have the potential to coalesce into more enduring trait-level changes (Hudson & Fraley, 2018).

Imagery rescripting

Imagery rescripting is an experiential therapeutic technique that uses imagery and imagination to intervene in traumatic memories. It consists of prompting patients to *rescript* the autobiographical memory in line with their unmet needs. The process is guided by a therapist who works with the client to define ways to work with particular trauma memories, images, or nightmares (Arntz, 2012). Clients are guided to recall memories of trauma from the field vantage point as an exposure component. With the help of the therapists, the client changes the imagery to script a different outcome. The purpose is to gain mastery over the difficult image. It may involve regaining control over the event, creating new outcomes, or re-establishing power over the narrative of the event. This can address client's unmet core needs resulting from the memory/experience (Hackmann, 2011). It is practiced in three steps: 1) Imagine the traumatic event in detail, 2) imagine the client or someone else intervenes and changes the outcome, and 3) imagine the client receiving comfort or reassurance (Holmes et al., 2007).

Adaptive disclosure

Adaptive disclosure (AD: Litz et al., 2016) is an eight-session treatment that was designed for military marines with PTSD stemming from a variety of traumatic deployment experiences. The approach combines imaginal exposure to activate trauma-related emotions and uses cognitive and experiential techniques to modify maladaptive thoughts, beliefs and interpretations of their combat and operational experiences. It addresses traumas such as threat of life, traumatic loss and grief, and moral injury. Moral injury includes experiences that violate closely held moral beliefs and ethic codes (Gray et al., 2021). This is particularly related to concerns of self-blame which may be accurate once out of the circumstances but disrupts post-deployment adjustment. AD helps people recommit to their pre-event personal ethical and moral standards.

Adaptive disclosure as a therapeutic strategy is described in three steps: (1) In an intake session, information about the presenting problem is gathered, the case is conceptualized and categorized in one of the three stress categories (i.e., fear-based stress, loss related stress, or moral injury), and the treatment plan is clarified. (2) The next six sessions provide psychoeducation and incorporate imaginal exposure exercises (20–30 minutes of exposure) to facilitate emotional processing of deployment experiences, to reveal associations and beliefs about meaning and implications of their experiences. The imagery exposure and meaning making is tailored to the type of event experienced. The service member or veteran recalls details of the event (exposure) and then processes their reactions including implications, why it is difficult, grief or guilt, and cognitive distortions such as all-or-nothing thinking. They may also use the empty chair technique to deliver communications to a relevant person (What would you like to say? What would they say to you?). (3) The last session is used to review the experiences, underscore positive lessons learned, and plan for the future in light of what was addressed and achieved in the previous sessions. AD is accumulating supportive empirical evidence of effectiveness (Gray et al., 2012).

Comparing imagery-based treatments and holographic reprocessing

Similar to these approaches, holographic reprocessing addresses emotional and interpersonal patterns, repeating themes, or issues that have not been fully processed. Like the other treatments, holographic reprocessing uses imagery to help connect to deeper emotional issues and associations. In all of these treatments, imagery is used as a source of delivering comfort to one's younger self.

Unlike other treatments, holographic reprocessing is not exposure-based or a desensitization procedure. Participants do not have to relive past traumas in detail, nor does the trauma experience need to be activated. The trauma event is not avoided, but rather it is not activated for the purpose of desensitization. Holographic reprocessing also does not engage the therapist as an object for re-enacting patterns, nor is used specifically as the source of re-parenting.

One distinction from the others is that holographic reprocessing uses strategies to consider context, and alternative perspectives to shift meaning and understanding. It seeks meta-reframes by broadening one's perception.

This step is not included in any of the other treatments. In AD, meaning may be addressed as part of the conversation, but it is restructured from a cognitive-behavioral perspective. However, holographic reprocessing helps people consider events from the observer perspective, outside of oneself, to consider context.

Chapter summary

Holographic reprocessing is similar to and distinct from several accepted, evidence-based treatments. This chapter outlined these similarities and differences. Several unique factors are addressed through holographic reprocessing including developing coping skills, addressing patterns, and considering context and meaning.

Chapter 14

Current outcome research

This chapter presents findings of 25 outcome studies examining holographic reprocessing and warrior renew treatments.

Holographic reprocessing outcome studies

As mentioned in the Preface, 25 outcome studies have been conducted to date: 17 outcome studies on holographic reprocessing and eight studies on warrior renew treatment. These have demonstrated effective use of these treatments with a variety of people who have experienced various types of traumas. This includes survivors of sexual trauma across the lifespan including childhood and military, military combat, women going through divorce, cancer patients, those in substance abuse rehabilitation, and those with a recent suicide attempt. Although there are no studies, holographic reprocessing was recommended for those with eating disorders (Rivinius, 2013). It has been successfully used with racially diverse populations, gender-inclusive populations, inclusive of sexual orientation, adolescents, adults, military, and civilian populations. It has not only been effective in the United States, but also with diverse populations in Iran.

While having independent researchers conduct clinical trials accelerates the knowledge base without bias, it runs the risk of infidelity to the treatment model. Katz and colleagues have run ten studies. These should have good fidelity, but they run the risk of potential bias. However, with the accumulation of studies that find similar results, it reduces the likelihood that the results are due to chance. Research to date includes 14 randomized clinical trials, including comparisons with evidence-based treatments CPT, PE, and dialectic behavioral therapy (DBT: Linehan, 1993), with strong positive results (non-inferior to gold standard treatments and superior to control groups, all with low dropout rates) (Basharpoor et al., 2011; Katz et al., 2014a; Salehi et al., 2019). It was found that holographic reprocessing decreased symptoms of anxiety, depression, PTSD, and negative cognitions. Holographic reprocessing also improved positive factors such as optimism, self-esteem, and cognitive flexibility, and increased a fighting spirit in cancer patients. Table 14.1 is a summary of the 17 outcome studies testing holographic reprocessing.

DOI: 10.4324/9781003223429-17

Table 14.1 Summary of 17 outcome studies on holographic reprocessing

Reference	Sample	Outcome
Katz et al. (2008)	17 women veterans with sexual trauma PTSD, pre-post-treatment design	Significant reduction in negative cognitions, with large effect sizes and 47% with reliable change, 0 dropout
Basharpoor et al. (2011)*	60 male adolescents with mixed trauma, randomly assigned to HR, CPT, and control group	Active treatments were superior to control group on reducing negative cognitions. HR: stronger in reducing self-blame than CPT
Narimani et al. (2011)* Narimani et al. (2013)*	60 male adolescents with mixed trauma, randomly assigned to HR, CPT, and control group	HR was superior to CPT in reducing anxiety, dissociation, and PTSD symptoms, while CPT was superior in reducing depression
Katz et al. (2014b)*	51 women veterans with military sexual trauma were randomly assigned to HR, PE, or present centered therapy	Active treatments were superior to control group but not different than each other on PTSD, anxiety, or depression, negative cognitions. HR had significantly lower dropout than PE
Otared et al. (2016)	3 male veterans with PTSD had 9 sessions of HR with pre- and post-treatment and 1 month follow-up assessments	All had reduced arousal and intrusion, maintained at follow-up. Noted a change in clients' perceptions of traumatic event, themselves, and others. It is through this perceptual shift they were able to gain new insight
Mehrparvar et al. (2017)*	30 women with cancer were randomly assigned to HR or control group, HR received nine 60-min sessions	HR improved mental adjustment to cancer: improved fighting spirit scores, decreased scores of helpless/hopelessness, anxious preoccupation, but not fatalism or cognitive avoidance
Kasai et al. (2018)*	30 women who applied to the court for divorce were randomly assigned to HR vs control	HR decreased intrusive memories, inability to control emotions, depression, negative traumatic cognitions about self, world, and self-blame
Rezapour & Zakeri (2019)	2 depressed women, had 12 sessions of HR with pre- and post-treatment and 1- and 2-month follow-up assessments	Statistical and clinically meaningful reduction of rumination and fear of negative evaluation, and improved meaning of life, sustained at follow-up

Reference	Sample	Outcome
Salehi et al. (2019a)*	30 women applicants for divorce faced with infidelity were randomly assigned to HR vs control group	HR improved affective control and emotion regulation
Narimani et al. (2019)*	30 Female divorce applicants referred to Bijar County Court in 2015–2016 were randomly assigned to HR vs control group	HR improved women's general health and cognitive emotion regulation compared to control condition
Salehi et al. (2019b)*	45 depressed patients with recent suicide attempt were assigned randomly into three groups HR, dialectical behavior therapy (DBT), and control group (15 cases per group).	Both active treatments were superior to control, HR and DBT improved cognitive flexibility equally, DBT improved impulsivity more than HR
Salehi & Beshlideh (2020)*	Depressive patients with attempted Suicide, 30 participants were selected through a simple random sampling and assigned randomly into HR and control groups	HR increased cognitive flexibility, affective control and social adjustment more than control ($p<.000$)
Salehi et al. (2020)*	Depressed women who attempted suicide. 30 were randomly assigned to HR or control group (15 each)	HR was associated with improved emotion regulation, and decreased impulsivity compared to the control group ($p<.000$)
Salehi et al. (2020)*	45 depressed patients who attempted suicide were randomly assigned to HR, DBT, and control groups (15 each)	HR, DBT improved affect control and social adjust more than control group. HR improved social adjustment more than DBT
Aghajani et al. (2021)*	30 women with breast cancer who had mastectomy were selected and randomly divided into the experimental and control groups (15 each). The experimental group, while receiving pharmacotherapy, collectively underwent holographic reprocessing therapy in 9 one-hour sessions (two sessions per week) for 5 weeks; however, the control group received only pharmacotherapy	HR was associated with significantly increased cognitive flexibility and posttraumatic growth compared to control group
Eftekhari et al. (2022)*	30 screened with PTSD were randomly assigned to HR or wait list control group (15 each)	HR improved avoidance, intrusions, and hyperarousal symptoms of PTSD

Note: HR = holographic reprocessing, * = randomized controlled trial.

References listed in Appendix A.

In addition, holographic reprocessing is the basis for the group treatment program, *warrior renew* (Katz, 2014) a transdiagnostic protocol designed to treat common issues associated with sexual trauma for gender-inclusive populations. It is typically delivered in a group format which helps address stigma and isolation by providing social support. It is designed to help participants manage anxiety triggers, as well as self-blame, anger and resentment due to injustice and lack of closure, and examines the impact on interpersonal functioning.

Of the eight published outcome studies on warrior renew (Table 14.2), six were conducted with women veterans within the Department of Veterans Affairs (VA) medical settings. These pragmatic trials demonstrated significant decreased symptoms of PTSD, anxiety, and depression, and increased positive factors such as self-esteem, optimism, and secure attachment, with large effect sizes and low dropout rates (Katz et al., 2014b; Katz et al., 2016; Katz, 2016; Katz & Sawyer, 2020). Initially developed as a 12-week study, a brief 8-week version showed strong efficacy in a study of 30 female veterans who demonstrated significant improvements (Katz & Sawyer, 2020). A longitudinal trial of 32 female veterans demonstrated sustained improvements twelve months from baseline (Katz et al., 2015). Participants in these studies had multiple social, mental, and physical health challenges including dual diagnoses, chronic illness, chronic pain, and homelessness, demonstrating the treatment modality's effectiveness in complex, real-world veteran populations. Similar results were found with non-veteran women in a residential substance abuse treatment program (Hemma et al., 2018). The treatment was also delivered in novel formats including a five-day retreat (Katz & Jensen, 2022), and over video teleconferencing (Katz, 2023.

Change on the PTSD Checklist (PCL) (Weathers et al., 1993) and PTSD Checklist for DSM-V (PCL-5) (Weathers et al., 2013) demonstrated significant improvements in five trials with female veterans conducted at the VA with medium to large effect sizes across all of these trials (effect sizes ranging from .59 to 2.07). Figure 14.1 shows a graph depicting change scores on the PCL and PCL-5 for these studies.

The eight studies had low attrition rates (percentages: 13, 10, 11, 21, 65, 21, 0, 30). The high rate in the substance abuse program included everyone who enrolled in the program. They had a high attrition rate in general, and the addition of warrior renew increased retention with graduates reporting a 95% reliable change score. One explanation for the high retention across the studies may be that warrior renew has an emphasis on community-building and improving interpersonal attachment as was found in the Katz et al. (2016) study. Participant comments in various trials provided consistent reports that the group process enhanced supportive bonds with each other. Even those who were initially worried about engaging in a group, stated they enjoyed the comradery and peer support. In addition, participants

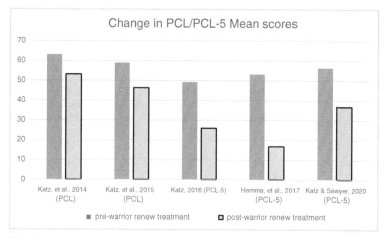

Change in PCL/PCL-5 Mean scores

pre-warrior renew treatment   post-warrior renew treatment

PCL= Posttraumatic checklist for DSM IV, PCL-5 Posttraumatic checklist for DSM-5

Figure. 14.1 Change in PCL/PCL-5 mean scores in five studies of warrior renew. PCL= Posttraumatic Checklist for DSM IV, PCL-5 Posttraumatic Checklist for DSM-5

Table 14.2 Summary of eight studies on warrior renew

	Treatment format/ reference	Sample size of women with sexual trauma (% dropout)	Statistically significant outcomes
Katz et al. (2014a)	12-week VA Intensive Outpatient Program (IOP) 5 days/week	119 enrolled, 97 completed (13%)	Decreased PTSD, anxiety, depression, negative thinking, and increased self-esteem, optimism. RC: 60%
Katz et al. (2015)	12-week IOP at VA, followed from baseline to 12-months	41 enrolled, 37 completed treatment (10%), 30 completed study 12 months from baseline (27%)	Sustained decreased PTSD symptoms, depression, anxiety, negative thinking. Improved quality of life at 12 months. RC: 70%
Katz et al. (2016)	12-week VA IOP	75 enrolled, 62 completed (11%)	Improved perceived secure attachment, decreased insecure attachment
Katz (2016)	VA outpatient, 12-week group meeting 2 times a week	43 enrolled, 34 completed (21%)	Decreased PTSD, negative thinking, anxiety, depression, and increased self-esteem, optimism. RC: 75%

	Treatment format/ reference	Sample size of women with sexual trauma (% dropout)	Statistically significant outcomes
Hemma et al. (2018)	60-day community residential substance abuse program	55 enrolled, 19 completed (65%)	Decreased PTSD, anxiety depression, and increased self-esteem, optimism. RC: 95%
Katz & Sawyer (2020)	VA Primary Care, Brief Warrior Renew (8 sessions)	38 enrolled, 30 completed (21%)	Decreased PTSD, anxiety, depression, and increased, self-esteem, optimism. RC: 73%
Katz & Jensen (2022)	5-day retreat for veterans at Omega Institute of Holistic Studies	20 enrolled, 20 completed the retreat (0%)	Decreased anxiety, depression, and improved negative thinking (very large effect sizes)
Katz (2023)	Brief Warrior Renew (8 sessions) delivered over video teleconferencing for women veterans during COVID-19 pandemic	40 enrolled, 28 completed (30%) (7.5% dropped due to internet connectivity)	80% stated they preferred virtual format, 20% did not; decreased depression, anxiety, and negative thinking

Note: RC = Percentage of sample with reliable clinical change on the Posttraumatic Cognitions Inventory (PTCI) measuring negative thinking. Reliable change means the outcome finding is above what could be expected by chance based on the reliability of a particular measure. This was at the 95% confidence interval.

References listed in Appendix A.

stated they appreciated learning about why they have their reactions and felt the class content was particularly helpful.

Summary of research findings

Consistent across these clinical trials, findings support that holographic reprocessing is associated with significant decreases in symptoms of PTSD, anxiety, depression, negative thinking, particularly self-blame, and improvements in cognitive flexibility, social adjustment, emotion regulation, fighting spirit, posttraumatic growth, optimism, secure attachment, self-esteem, and quality of life. Many of these findings were superior to minimal treatment control groups and some factors superior to evidence-based treatments. However, more research is needed including large randomized controlled trails, and with a larger pool of clinicians conducting the studies. For Warrior Renew, more diverse samples are also needed. Nonetheless, a growing body of outcome research supports the promising efficacy of holographic reprocessing in diverse populations delivered in a variety of formats by diverse clinicians.

Appendix A: Publications related to holographic reprocessing and warrior renew

Publications related to holographic reprocessing

Holographic reprocessing outcome studies, chronological

Katz, L. S., Snetter, M. R., Robinson, A. H., Hewitt, P., & Cojucar, G. (2008). Holographic reprocessing: Empirical evidence to reduce posttraumatic cognitions in women veterans with PTSD from sexual trauma and abuse. *Psychotherapy: Theory, Research, Practice, Training, 45*(2), 186–198. https://doi.org/10.1037/0033-3204.45.2.186.

Basharpoor, S., Narimani, M., Gamari-Givev, H., Abolgasemi, A., & Molavi, P. (2011). Effect of cognitive processing therapy and holographic reprocessing on reduction of posttraumatic cognitions in students exposed to trauma. *Iran Journal Psychiatry, 6*(4),138–144. PMID: 22952539; PMCID: PMC3395960.

Narimani, M., Basharpoor, S., Gamari-Givi, H., & Abolgasemi, A. (2011). Effectiveness of cognitive processing therapy and holographic reprocessing on the reduction of psychological symptoms in students exposed to trauma. *Journal of Clinical Psychology, 3*(11), 41–53.

Narimani, M., Basharpoor, S., Gamarigive, H., & Abolgasemi, A. (2013). Impact of cognitive processing and holographic reprocessing on posttraumatic symptoms improvement amongst Iranian students. *Advances in Cognitive Science, 15*(2[58]), 50–62.

Katz, L. S., Douglas, S., Zaleski, K. L., Williams, J., Huffman, C., & Cojucar, G. (2014b). Comparing holographic reprocessing and prolonged exposure for women veterans with sexual trauma: A pilot randomized trial. *Journal of Contemporary Psychotherapy, 44*, 9–19.

Otared, N, Borjali, A. Sohrabi, F., & Basharpoor, S. (2016). Efficacy of holographic reprocessing on arousal and intrusion symptoms in veterans with posttraumatic stress disorder. *Studies in Medical Sciences, 27*(5), 427–437

Mehrparvar, S., Hajloo, N., & Aboolghasemi, A. (2017). The effectiveness of Holographic Reprocessing Therapy on mental adjustment to cancer in women with cancer. *Studies in Medical Sciences, 28*(5), 343–352. http://umj.umsu.ac.ir/article-1-3923-en.html.

Kasai N., Narimani, M., & Basharpoor, S. (2018). The effectiveness of holographic reprocessing therapy in improving traumatic memories and post-traumatic cognitions of women claiming divorce. *Counseling Journal*, 15(61), 35–37.

Rezapour, M., & Zakeri, M. (2019). The effectiveness of holographic re-treatment on the meaning of life, fear of negative evaluation and rumination of depressed women. *Counseling Culture and Psychotherapy*, 10(3900588), 49–70.

Salehi, M., Naami, A., & Kazemi, N. (2019a). Effectiveness of holographic reprocessing on affective control and difficulty in emotion regulating of women applicants for the divorce faced with infidelity. *Journal Quarterly Journal of Women and Society*, 9(36), 197–216

Narimani, M., Kazemi, N., & Basharpoor, S. (2019). The effectiveness of holographic reprocessing on general health and cognitive emotion regulation in female divorce applicants referred to Bijar County court in 2015–2016: An educational trial. *Journal of Rafsanjan University of Medical Sciences and Health Services*, 18(3), 237–250.

Salehi, M., Hamid, N., Beshlideh, K., & Arshadi, N. (2019b). Comparison of the effectiveness of holographic reprocessing and dialectical behavioral therapy on cognitive flexibility and impulsivity among depressed patients with a suicide attempt in Ilam, Iran. *Journal of Ilam University of Medical Sciences*, 27(5) 1–14. https://doi.org/doi:10.29252/sjimu.27.5.1.

Salehi, M., & Beshlideh, K. (2020). The effectiveness of holographic reprocessing therapy on cognitive flexibility, affective control and social adjustment on depressive patients with attempted suicide in Ilam City. *Counseling Culture and Psychotherapy*, 11(43), 183–216. https://doi.org/10.22054/qccpc.2020.50615.2338.

Salehi, M., Beshlideh, K., & Kazemzade, K. (2020). Effectiveness of holographic reprocessing therapy on cognitive emotion regulation strategies and impulsivity of women attempted suicide in Ilam City. *Quarterly Journal of Women and Society*, 11, e17192. https://doi.org/1001.1.20088566.1399.11.43.9.7.

Aghajani, S., Khoshsorour, S., & Taghizadeh Hir, S. (2021). The effectiveness of holographic reprocessing therapy on cognitive flexibility and posttraumatic growth in women with breast cancer. Journal Arak University Medical Science, 24(1). http://jams.arakmu.ac.ir/article-1-6471-en.html.

Eftekhari A., Bakhtiari M., & Arani A. M. (2022). The effectiveness of holographic reprocessing therapy (HR) on the avoidance, intrusions and hyperarousal symptoms in PTSD patients. *Medical Science*, 26, e2024.

Other publications on holographic reprocessing

Katz, L. S. (2001). Holographic reprocessing: A cognitive-experiential psychotherapy. *Psychotherapy: Theory, Research, Practice, Training*, 38(2), 186–197. https://doi.org/10.1037/0033-3204.38.2.186.

Katz, L. S. (2005). *Holographic reprocessing: A cognitive-experiential psychotherapy for the treatment of trauma.* New York: Brunner-Routledge.
Katz, L. (2007). What is Holographic Reprocessing? Los Angeles Psychologist, Sept/Oct.
Katz, L. (2019). Holographic reprocessing couple therapy with military couples. In P. Pitta & C. Datchi (Eds.), *Integrative couple and family therapy: Treatment models for complex clinical issues.* Washington DC: American Psychological Association.

Publications related to warrior renew

Warrior renew outcome studies

Katz, L., Cojucar, G., Douglas, S., & Huffman, C. (2014a). Renew: An integrative psychotherapy program for women Veterans with sexual trauma. *Journal of Contemporary Psychotherapy, 44*(3), 163–171.
Katz, L. Cojucar, G., Hoff, R., Lindl, C., Huffman, C. & Drew, T. (2015). Longitudinal outcomes of Renew: A sexual trauma treatment program for women Veterans. *Journal of Contemporary Psychotherapy, 45*(3), 143–150.
Katz, L. (2016). Efficacy of Warrior Renew group therapy for female veterans who have experienced military sexual trauma. *Psychological Services, 13*(4), 364–372.
Katz, L., Park, S., Cojucar, G., Huffman, C, & Douglas, S. (2016). Improved attachment style for female veterans who graduated Warrior Renew sexual trauma treatment. *Violence and Victims, 31*(4), 680–691.
Hemma, G., McNab, A., & Katz, L. (2018). Efficacy of sexual trauma treatment in a substance abuse residential program for women. *Journal of Contemporary Psychotherapy, 48*(1), 1–8, https://doi.org/10.1007/s10879–017–9365–8
Katz, L. S., & Sawyer, W. N. (2020). Pragmatic trial of brief Warrior Renew group therapy for military sexual trauma in VA primary care. *Psychological Services, 17*(4), 433–442. https://doi.org/10.1037/ser0000325
Katz, L., & Jensen, G. (2022). Outcomes of a five-day therapeutic retreat to reduce symptoms related to military sexual trauma using the Warrior Renew program. *Journal of Contemporary Psychotherapy, 52*, 311–318. https://doi.org/10.1007/s10879-022-09545-8
Katz, L. S. (2023). Delivering brief warrior renew over video teleconferencing to women veterans with military sexual trauma: A pragmatic trial. *Psychological Services.* Advance online publication. https://doi.org/10.1037/ser0000786.

Other publications related to warrior renew

Katz, L. (2014). *Warrior renew: Healing military sexual trauma.* New York: Springer.

Other publications related to military sexual trauma

Katz, L., Cojucar, G., Beheshti, S., Nakamura, E., & Murray, M. (2012). Military sexual trauma during combat: Prevalence, readjustment, and gender differences in those deployed in the conflicts in Iraq and Afghanistan. *Violence and Victims, 27*(4), 487–499.

Zaleski, K., & Katz, L. (2014) Alice in Wonderland: Exploring the experience of female services members with a pregnancy resulting from rape. *Social Work in Mental Health, 12,* 391–410.

Pence, P., Katz, L., Huffman, C., & Cojucar, G. (2014). Delivering Integrative Restoration-yoga Nidra meditation (iRest) to women with sexual trauma at a veteran's medical center: A pilot study. *International Journal of Yoga Therapy,* (24), 53–62.

Katz, L. (2015). *Treating military sexual trauma.* New York: Springer.

Katz, L. Huffman, C., & Cojucar, G. (2016). In her own words: Semi-structured interviews of women veterans who experienced military sexual trauma. *Journal of Contemporary Psychotherapy, 47*(3), 181–189.

Appendix B: Therapist handouts

Checklist of skills, metaphors, and strategies to use in holographic reprocessing

Epstein's cognitive-experiential theory

1   Cognitive and experiential systems
2   Tree falling in the forest
3   Buying a car
4   Jellybean experiment

Metaphors for explaining rationale for holographic reprocessing

5   String of holiday lights
6   Address the blueprint not the houses
7   What does your future look like if you are living from the past?
8   Driving while focusing on the rear-view mirror, or driving with the emergency brake on
9   Wearing virtual reality goggles

Emotion regulation skills

10   Emotions flow through us like water flows through a hose
11   Signal/cleansing breaths
12   Grounding through one's senses, slow deep breathing, attention to one's feet
13   What-is… thinking (instead of what-if… thinking)
14   Positive focal point
15   Calming hand poses
16   COPE strategy
17   Washing machine metaphor

Experiential hologram discovery/mapping patterns

18   Interpersonal experiential hologram inventory
19   Gendlin's focusing on body sensation, listening to intuition
20   Journaling about relationships
21   Pot on the stove template (a collaborative process to define components)

Types of experiential holograms

22   Interpersonal patterns of being neglected, rejected, betrayed, endangered
23   Moral injury
24   Victim of a crime or attack
25   Complicated grief
26   Surviving a life-threatening experience

Metaphors for seeing context

27   Field mouse vs observing eagle (observer vantage point)
28   Tissue box (multiple truths) Considering agenda, motivation from other's point of view
29   Age comparison (perspective of age)
30   Book of norm (your assumptions and expectations may not be what other people think)
31   Hindsight advantage (knowing the outcome)

Meta-reframes

32   Seeking explanations and meaning from a broad perspective
33   Children are meant to evolve past their parents
34   Connecting dots: seeing how a negative event might have led to something positive

Metaphors for disengaging and accepting

35   Poetic justice (to release anger/resentment, injustice)
36   Blue pen (acceptance of what is)
37   It takes a thief for a theft to occur (to release self-blame)
38   Shrinking machine (reducing fear)
39   Catcher's mitt (tossing back something that is not yours)

Letters

40   Letter to one's younger self
41   Letter to someone who died
42   Letter to one's future self

Imagery reprocessing

43   Observer vantage point training: recalling a bite of food
44   What would you say? Offering compassion, understanding, not your fault
45   What would you do? Offer a gift, hug, take younger self out of a situation
46   Imagery to release deceased (seeing them as safe, happy, and free)
47   Imagery after surviving a near-death event (telling younger self you're going to be ok)

Post-traumatic growth

48   Commitment to actions of reparation post-moral injury
49   Mining golden nuggets along the path (any positives that came from the experience?)
50   Yes-attitude (while keeping no in your pocket)
51   Imagining meeting one's future self

Six steps for Implementing holographic reprocessing

These can be tailored to the needs of a client. Some may complete a step in one session while others may need more time.

- **Step 1: Introduction to treatment**

Learn more about trauma experience.
Explain cognitive-experiential theory (two systems, share the example of a tree falling in the forest).
Treatment addresses patterns (the blueprints not individual houses).
Teach skills: signal breath, cleansing breath or both.

- **Step 2: Emotion regulation skills**

Explain how emotions organize our memories (string of holiday lights). Neural networks are formed to be adaptive as protective against threat or danger.
Address emotions: anxiety and triggers/discuss what triggers client, and/or anger via poetic justice, distraction/shift attention.
Teach skills: COPE, washing machine metaphor, slow deep breathing, aromatherapy, grounding.

- **Step 3: Identify experiential hologram**

Discuss holograms and experiential holograms as implicit perceptions of reality playing in the background – like wearing virtual reality goggles, that filter how you anticipate, perceive, and react to life events.
Engage in experiential discovery, writing exercises, interpersonal experiential hologram inventory. Pot on the stove to map interpersonal experiential hologram.
Teach coping skills such as the positive focal point, and calming hand poses coupled with slow deep breathing.

- **Step 4: Discuss context**

Consider past from a new perspective: Observer vantage point (eagle, field mouse).
Could also include: Tissue box for multiple truths, Age comparison, It takes a thief (e.g., dislodging self-blame), Hindsight advantage, and Meta-reframes. Consider different points of view to understand and make meaning of the experience.
With new knowledge, what would you say to your younger self? Homework: write letter.

- ### *Step 5: Imagery reprocessing*

Preparation: Choose who to visit: training on observer vantage point (bite of food exercise). Explain rationale/expectations for imagery reprocessing; identify what to say or do if client met younger self, or visit image of deceased from an observer vantage point.
Implement: Imagery reprocessing exercise.

- ### *Step 6: Integration and moving forward*

Visioning the future: What's important, shift focus towards future; handling potential relapse of old hologram, embracing a new self-defined identity, consider opening to new experiences consistent with values, and goals.

INTAKE ASSESSMENT

Confidentiality Statement & Informed Consent
Chief Complaint:
History of Presenting Issue:
Current Life Circumstances:

Sleep
Relationships/supportive others:
Employment current/history:
Current housing:
Legal issues:
Activities/hobbies/exercise

History of Substance Use:

Tobacco, alcohol, marijuana, other drugs (amphetamines, cocaine, benzodiazepines, opioids), caffeine

Childhood History:

Trauma History:

Childhood abuse, trauma, or hardships?
History of perpetrating abuse or harming others?
Other traumatic or life-threatening experiences (abuse, harassment, military experiences, accidents, medical, losses, natural disasters)?

Mental Status:

Oriented, appearance and behavior, mood, speech, thought content, thought process, capacity for insight, judgment, memory

Assessment Inventories:

Safety and Risk Screening:

Administer suicide risk screen, assess for safety issues (homicide risk, intimate partner violence, access to firearms). Positive screens need follow-up assessment and safety plans

Suicide Risk Assessment:

[ ] **High risk:** Requires psychiatric stabilization
[ ] **Intermediate risk:** Chronic suicidal ideation, but not acute risk. Currently stable
[ ] **Low risk:** Current risk minimal. Periodic reassessment at follow-up appointments

TYPES OF HOLOGRAMS (focus of treatment)

[ ] **Interpersonal pattern** (e.g., of being neglected, rejected, betrayed, endangered)

[ ] **Victim of trauma** (self-blame, disbelief/intrusive thoughts, fear)

[ ] **Moral injury** (guilt, self-blame or self-loathing, remorse, intrusive thoughts)

[ ] **Grief** (sadness, guilt, disbelief/intrusive thoughts, regrets)

Does the therapist believe holographic reprocessing is appropriate for client?

If not, pursue appropriate plan

If so, explain treatment, assess if holographic reprocessing is welcomed/good fit for client. Present the rationale and what they can expect (informed consent)

Participants will be:

- Learning emotion regulation skills
- Identifying their experiential holograms
- Discussing different ways to make sense of the past using a variety of tools
- Engaging in imagery reprocessing to get closure and completion of past trauma

Key points that can be used to explain this approach. (Therapist chooses what to share to help client understand the reasoning and goals of the treatment during intake. The rest can be explained in subsequent sessions as appropriate.)

- Cognitive experiential theory (two systems, use example of tree falling in the forest)
- Emotions connect memories like a string of holiday lights metaphor
- For interpersonal trauma: In this treatment, we don't focus on specific events of trauma but rather we address the underlying core issues. We address relationship blueprints not the houses (or relationships) constructed from the blueprint
- The past is influencing their life. This is like driving while focusing on rearview mirror. It is difficult to move forward when their attention is stuck in the past
- Or: When there is something unresolved from the past, it is like trying to drive with the emergency brake on

Scripts for emotion regulation

Signal breath script

"The signal breath goes like this, take a deep breath in through the nose holding it for 5 seconds and then exhale through the mouth. It's based on the principle that you can't be relaxed and tense at the same time. It's like having either an open fist or a closed fist. It's one or the other... so when you're holding the breath, you're intensifying the tension and then when you release the breath you get a nice deep relaxation. One of the ways to remember this, is think of a signal light. We stop at a red light (holding the breath) and then go at the green light (exhale). This signals the body that it's time to relax. So, let's practice this together. Okay, get comfortable and we're going to inhale through the nose, hold it at the top... and then release through the mouth. Good! let's try that one more time, signal breath: deep breath in through the nose, hold it at the top 1 2 3 4 5, and then release through the mouth. Signaling the body, it's time to relax."

Cleansing breath script

"The cleansing breath is an easy technique—it is simply a deep breath in through the nose and out with a sigh... Imagine cleansing away all of your stress when you exhale. You can even imagine the breath is like a waterfall washing away the stress. There are several benefits of this breath: It helps kick in the inhibitory system or the parasympathetic system to help you parachute down from stress. It also helps by opening the throat and chest which can get tight when you feel angry, anxious, or intimidated. When you sigh, feel your shoulders releasing, and your mind and body resetting."

Grounding script

"Grounding is a helpful strategy when you're feeling anxious, uneasy, worried, spacey, or just not feeling centered in your body. With grounding you're literally going to ground your energy to the earth by focusing on your feet. Feel your feet, wiggle your toes, and feel your feet pressing into the floor. You can imagine strings of energy connecting the soles of your feet to the center of the earth. Feeling gravity supporting you. We're grounding your energy just like grounding an electronic device by sending the electricity to the earth, this keeps the device safe, and prevents power surges. Similarly, we are doing the same thing with our bodies, by connecting through the feet to the earth. Perhaps you can find an opportunity to walk barefoot on some sand or grass or maybe even lie down on the ground and feel your whole body connecting to the earth. Simply being out in nature can be grounding, and helps you reset your mood, energy, and mental well-being. This can include walking in a park or forest or going to a beach or waterfront area. Being around trees or water and breathing in fresh air can be very grounding."

"You can also practice the grounding breath. When we're anxious, we tend to have shallow quick breaths, and when we're more relaxed and grounded we have slower deeper breaths. So, what you want to do is slow down your breathing... slow inhale through the nose and slowly exhale through the mouth. To assist, you can synchronize your arm movements with the breath. On the inhale, lift your arms up and on the exhale lower the arms down, matching breath with movement. So, let's try that, inhale, lifting arm up and exhaling lowering the arms down for the grounding breath.... A couple of other grounding tips: be mindful of eating sugar and caffeine as these will make you feel more anxious and uneasy. Instead, a little protein is grounding and drinking water helps restore balance to the body."

Script: Calming hand pose palms together

"This exercise is very easy and it helps calm the nervous system. What you're going to do is put your palms together. This is also called the prayer pose. Place your thumbs at the center of your chest. This is called the heart center. Then extend the space between your fingers so your pinkies face outward towards the center of the room. Holding this position and breathe. You can keep your eyes open or closed. Breathing slowly... feeling the calming and balancing nature of holding your palms together."

Script: Calming hand pose chest and belly

"In this exercise, you can start by rubbing your hands together to create some heat and then place one hand on your chest, and the other on your belly region, palms facing towards the body. Feel the warmth of your hands going into your body. Hold the pose and breathe. This is used for comfort, soothing, and calming. It is particularly good for grief."

Note: people can choose which ever hand (right or left) they want to place on the chest or belly region.

Script: Resetting and regulating one's nervous system

"Find a comfortable place to sit or lie down, feeling supported by whatever is beneath you. If you are sitting in a chair, make sure your back is supported and your feet are on the ground, or if you are lying down, maybe place a pillow under your neck and a pillow under your knees for extra support. Feel yourself settling into a place of ease. Bring your attention to your body. Feeling present in your body. Use a calming hand position, or let your hands rest comfortably in your lap or by your side. You can start with a signal breath, a deep breath in through the nose, hold it at the top (count to 4–5), and then exhale through the mouth. Focusing on your breath. Practice slow deep breathing extending the inhale and then extending the exhale. Slow even breaths. Staying present in the body. If you'd like, think of your positive focal point or any positive image or positive emotion, something that makes you feel good like appreciation, love, or something that brings you happiness. If you have trouble generating a positive feeling, think of an image or something that makes you smile (e.g., a pet, loved ones, being at the beach, or even a large hot fudge sundae!).... hold on to that feeling, growing it in your body, while letting the image fade away. Allow yourself to exhale completely, releasing any tension in your body. Maybe on the next exhale, notice your shoulders or chest release a bit more. Feeling your entire body melting into the chair or floor. Keeping your focus on being present and continue slow deep breathing. If a thought comes up, just let it pass by, like a cloud passing in the sky. And bring your attention back to this particular breath. This brand-new breath. Inhaling and exhaling. Enjoying this moment... and this brand-new breath. (*Pause*) Inhale opening to life, and exhale releasing all that no longer serves you. And we'll end with a cleansing breath. Take a deep breath in through the nose, and release with a sigh. And again, big breath in... stretching... yawning... inhale and exhale with a sigh."

Guided imagery (beach and forest scenes)

Script: Guided imagery beach scene

"This is a guided imagery to imagine going to a beautiful tropical beach. Find a place where you feel comfortable. If you are sitting in a chair, make sure your back is supported and your feet are on the ground, or if you are lying down, maybe place a pillow under your neck and a pillow under your knees for extra support. Let your body settle into a place of ease. Just let your body melt into whatever is supporting you. Arms resting comfortably in your lap or by your side. Let's start with the signal breath, deep breath in through the nose, hold it at the top... and then exhale through the mouth. Breathing nice and gently, inhaling and exhaling. Notice the subtle movement... with each inhale expanding and with each exhale releasing... just like the ocean – the waves coming up to shore... and then going back out to sea. Matching your breath with the waves of the ocean... inhaling the waves come to shore, and exhaling the waves go back out to sea. Watching the waves, rhythmically moving just like your breath. It's a beautiful day, the temperature is just right, warm and comfortable. The sky is clear and blue... maybe one small fluffy cloud in the distance. Listen to the sounds of the ocean, watching the waves going back and forth... and maybe you hear the call of a seagull in the distance. Feel a slight cool breeze from the fresh ocean air. You can smell the salt water in the air and maybe even taste it in the back of your throat. The water is so blue, almost a turquoise blue, just beautiful. Enjoy this moment at the beach, relaxing on the soft sand. Maybe you are lying down on the soft warm sand, or on a plush blanket or lounge chair, either way, you are completely supported and relaxed. Maybe wiggle your toes in the warm sand, or let the sand run through your fingers. Inhale as the waves come into shore, and exhale as they go back out to sea. Feel how your body feels when you are at the beach. Imagine feeling a sense of joy and well-being. Imagine your heart is smiling, your eyes are smiling, and your lips are smiling as you take in this moment. Let's take a deep breath of that beautiful fresh air with a little bit of saltiness to it, and then exhale out. Imagine as you breathe you are cleansing your mind and body. Refreshing your entire being—washing away all the stress. Feeling cleansed and refreshed. Let's end with a couple of cleansing breaths. Inhale through the nose, and exhale with a sigh. Wiggle your toes and your fingers. Let's take a deep breath in, opening your eyes, and exhale with a sigh... Stretching and yawning..."

Script: Guided imagery forest to a waterfall

"Settle into a place of ease, back against the chair, feet on the floor. If you are sitting in a chair, make sure your back is supported and your feet are on the ground, or if you are lying down, maybe place a pillow under your neck and a pillow under your knees for extra support. Let your body drop into a place of ease. Just let your body melt into whatever is supporting you. Arms resting comfortably in your lap or by your side. Let's start with the signal breath, deep breath in through the nose, hold it at the top... and then exhale through the mouth. Breathing nice and gently, inhaling and exhaling. Imagine walking on a path in the forest... on a dirt path, surrounded by tall evergreen trees. You can almost smell a hint of pine in the air, looking around seeing the trees, noticing the light as it finds its way through the branches. As you walk, you can hear the crunch of some leaves and pinecones beneath your feet. It's a beautiful day, clear blue sky, you can feel the warmth of the sun on your skin, continue walking on the path, surrounded by beautiful nature. Maybe you hear some birds in the distance. You look up and you see a little bird fly to a tree branch. Noticing the textured bark on the trees. Notice the ferns growing near the path and some large boulders. Walk around a boulder, and you notice you can easily climb to the top of the boulder and find a comfortable place to sit. From this perspective, you can see in the distance, a waterfall. Watch the water as it dances over the rocks and splashes up. Listening to the soothing sound of the waterfall. Imagine feeling cool and refreshed by the water splashing into the air. Breathe in the fresh air and imagine it is cleansing your mind and body. It's so peaceful being in the forest with the trees, and birds and the waterfall. Imagine feeling refreshed and relaxed. When you are ready, walk back along the forest path, noticing the trees, and finding yourself back in your chair (or where you lying down), feeling your body is grounded and supported. Let's take a cleansing breath: deep breath in through the nose, and out with a sigh. Slowly open your eyes, stretching your arms, and one more cleansing breath deep inhale through the nose out with a sigh. Stretching and yawning…"

Script: Body scan

"In this exercise, I will name each body part, sense what you feel, without judgment or needing to fix or change anything. Just notice it. Settle into a place of ease, back against the chair, feet on the floor. If you are sitting in a chair, make sure your back is supported and your feet are on the ground, or if you are lying down, maybe place a pillow under your neck and a pillow under your knees for extra support. Let your body settle into a place of ease. Just let your body melt into whatever is supporting you. Arms resting comfortably in your lap or by your side.

Let's start with the signal breath, deep breath in through the nose, hold it at the top... and then exhale through the mouth. Breathing nice and gently, inhaling and exhaling. Breathing normally. Good. Now we are going to do a body scan exercise to help you feel more grounded and relaxed. Let's start by bringing your awareness to your feet. Feel your feet on the ground, feel the soles of your feet connecting to the floor beneath you. Maybe wiggle your toes, feeling the tops of your feet, then the entire foot connecting to the earth. Your feet are anchoring you, grounding you, feeling solid. Now feel your ankles and then your calves also connected to your feet and to the ground. Feeling your knees... sensing your thighs. And breathing as you feel each part of your body. Feel yourself sitting on the chair, sinking into the chair, supporting your back and legs. Feel your back relaxing, your lower back and your upper back, as you let the chair hold and support you. Feel your arms and hands also supported —feeling heavier and relaxed. Sense your hands, imagine a ball of energy swirling in the palms of your hands, then all the way to your fingertips. Now tune into your shoulders. Feel your shoulders release a little more as you exhale... melting into the chair and becoming more relaxed. Notice your neck, the muscles that connect to your ears. Sense your outer ears, and feel the sensation of sound vibrating in your inner ears. Bring your attention to your eyes. Feel your eyelids, your eyeballs, and all the muscles around your eyes. Feel your forehead soften as you relax your eyes and your eyebrows. Notice your nose. Feel the air going in and out of your nostrils as you breathe. Feel your jaw, lips, and inside your mouth. Now bring your awareness to your entire body. Starting at the top of your head, scan your body from your head, neck, torso, down your arms to your hands and fingers, down your legs to your feet and the tips of your toes. Sensing your entire body. Being very present." (*Add optional mindfulness exercise here.*) "Ok, now we'll do a couple of cleansing breaths, deep breath in through the nose and out with a sigh. Opening your eyes... Stretching and yawning... deep breath in through the nose, and out with a sigh. Inhale opening to life, and exhale releasing all that no longer serves you."

Script: Imagery of hope

"Settle into a place of ease, back against the chair, feet on the floor. Let your body melt into the chair, arms resting comfortable in your lap or by your side. Let's start with the signal breath, deep breath in through the nose, hold it at the top... and then exhale through the mouth. Breathing nice and gently, inhaling and exhaling. Each breath is a brand-new experience. This particular breath, this inhale, this exhale. The breath moves through the body, and it passes, vanishes, dissolves like cotton candy. One breath goes, and another comes, sustaining life, keeping the body moving forward. Each individual breath is temporary and a moment in time, a fleeting experience. We cannot hold on to a breath, as much as we try, we have to let the breath go and move. The breath is moving through us. Similarly, our experiences, and life itself, moves through us. Once we understand that holding on does not serve us, we learn to open our grasp releasing all the tension, worries, fears, hurts, resentments... All that we've been holding and carrying, weighing us down. Like rising above it all, floating above the trees, looking down at the past, old thoughts, and feelings. Making room for new thoughts, feelings, experiences... Imagine releasing the past, and entering a new way of being that allows, surrenders, and opens to new, deeper, and more profound experiences. We may breathe more fully. Welcoming each breath as a brand-new experience. Being light, hollow, expansive. Creating room for laughter, connection, play, and joy. Inhale, opening to life, and exhale releasing all that no longer serves you. And a cleansing breath, inhale and exhale with a sigh. Feeling lighter and refreshed."

Script: for imagery reprocessing of an interpersonal experiential hologram

(*Note:* This uses a guided imagery along a country road. If this is a trigger for your client, do not use this image. Instead, use another image that is relaxing such as walking along a beach, or by a lake... do what is most comfortable for your client. Take your time when reading the script. Pause. Use a calm relaxing tone to your voice. Pay attention to your client's body language to monitor their reaction.)

"Ok, let's get started with a signal breath. Take a deep breath in through the nose, hold it at the top... and slowly exhale through the mouth. Good. Feel yourself sitting in your chair, your feet on the floor, and back supported by the chair. Feel your whole body supported by the chair beneath you. Let's take another signal breath, inhale through the nose... hold it at the top... and release through the mouth, releasing any tension in the body, melting into the chair beneath you. On the next exhale, relax your shoulders, and your chest... letting your arms and hands rest comfortably in your lap.... and breathing...

Now imagine walking on a country road. The sky is clear and blue. Maybe there is a small white cloud in the distance. It is a warm sunny day and you can feel the warmth of the sun on your skin. You can hear birds chirping in the trees. You are walking on a path lined with trees and flowers. The colors are vibrant and the air smells fresh and clean. Imagine walking on this beautiful day... allowing yourself to relax and take in this pleasant scene. Where are you on a scale of 1 to 10, where 10 is tense and 1 is very relaxed? Good. And notice with the next exhale you can go a bit deeper continuing to relax... breathing... bringing your level down just one notch at a time... Excellent... Up ahead you see a grassy clearing, approach the clearing. You can stop here for a while if you would like to continue to relax- maybe find a boulder that is smooth to the touch. You can sit on the fresh soft grass and lean against the boulder. Listening... perhaps you can hear a nearby stream bubbling, and birds chirping in the distance. Enjoy this moment, basking in the sun. Taking in all of the beauty of this scene. And breathe...

When you are ready, imagine that in the distance is the place where your younger self is. It may be hazy and far away. If you would like, imagine approaching the place as you, your current age self. You, right now, with all the knowledge and wisdom that you have gained up to this point of your life. Imagine there is a door. Approach the door and stop when you get in front of the door. Pause, breathe, know you are safe, and grounded. And when you are ready, imagine opening the door to your past...

Look around, can you see your younger self? What does your younger self look like, what is your younger self doing? Would you like to approach your younger self? What would you like to say? What does your younger self want or need to hear from you? (*Pause.*) Spend a moment talking to your younger self. (*Pause.*) Do you want to do anything? Does your younger self need anything from you—a hug or a special gift? (*Pause.*) Spend a moment giving your younger self what they need. (*Pause.*) Is there anything else you would like to say or do before you leave? (*Pause.*) Would you like to leave your younger self in the room or go somewhere else? (*Pause.*) Nod your head if you're ready to go. When you are ready and feel complete… imagine returning to the grassy clearing with the nearby stream… and then walking back on the country road… noticing the trees and flowers… breathing in the fresh air. Bring your awareness back to the room, sitting in the chair, feeling your body supported by the chair, feet on the ground. Let's take a cleansing breath, deep breath in through the nose and out of the mouth with a sigh. Slowly open your eyes, stretching and yawning. (*Take a few moments of silence.*)

How are you doing? What did you experience?"

Script: Imagery reprocessing of interpersonal experiential hologram with a message to one's future self

(This script can be modified if the client only wants to focus on meeting one's future self, imagine the door is to their future self, and substitute future self for younger self. If this is the case, then skip the message blown into the leaf.)

(*Note:* If a country road is a trigger, use another image that is relaxing such as walking along a beach. Take your time when reading the script. Pause. Use a calm relaxing tone to your voice. Pay attention to your client's body language to monitor their reactions.)

"Ok, let's get started with a signal breath. Take a deep breath in through the nose, hold it at the top… and slowly exhale through the mouth. Good. Feel yourself sitting in your chair, your feet on the floor, and back supported by the chair. Feel your whole body supported by the chair beneath you. Let's take another signal breath, inhale through the nose… hold it at the top… and release through the mouth, releasing any tension in the body, melting into the chair beneath you. On the next exhale, relax your shoulders, and your chest… letting your arms and hands rest comfortably in your lap…. and breathing…

Now imagine walking on a country road. The sky is clear and blue. Maybe there is a small white cloud in the distance. It is a warm sunny day and you can feel the warmth of the sun on your skin. You can hear birds chirping in the trees. You are walking on a path lined with trees and flowers. The colors are vibrant and the air smells fresh and clean. Imagine walking on this beautiful day… allowing yourself to relax and take in this pleasant scene. Where are you on a scale of 1 to 10, where 10 is tense and 1 is very relaxed? Good. And notice with the next exhale you can go a bit deeper continuing to relax... breathing... bringing your level down just one notch at a time... Excellent... Up ahead you see a grassy clearing, approach the clearing. You can stop here for a while if you would like to continue to relax- maybe find a boulder that is smooth to the touch. You can sit on the fresh soft grass and lean against the boulder. Listening... perhaps you can hear a nearby stream bubbling, and birds chirping in the distance. Enjoy this moment, basking in the sun. Taking in all of the beauty of this scene. And breathe...

When you are ready, imagine that in the distance is the place where your younger self is. It may be hazy and far away. If you would like, imagine approaching the place as you, your current age self. You, right now, with all the knowledge and wisdom that you have gained up to this point of your life. Imagine there is a door. Approach the door and stop when you get in front of the door. Pause, breathe, know you are safe, and grounded. And when you are ready, imagine opening the door to your past...

Look around, can you see your younger self? What does your younger self look like, what is your younger self doing? Would you like to approach your younger self? What would you like to say? What does your younger self want or need to hear from you? (*Pause.*) Spend a moment talking to your younger self. (*Pause.*) Do you want to do anything? Does your younger self need anything from you—a hug or a special gift? (*Pause.*) Spend a moment giving your younger self what they need. (*Pause.*) Is there anything else you would like to say or do before you leave? (*Pause.*) Would you like to leave your younger self in the room or go somewhere else? (*Pause.*) Nod your head if you're ready to go. When you are ready and feel complete...

Imagine returning to the grassy clearing with the nearby stream. Take a moment to pause here. Look for a leaf. Hold the leaf in your hands. Think of a message that you would like to send to your future self. (*Pause.*) blow your message into the leaf so that it is fused into the fibers. Then release the leaf into the stream. Imagine it floating to your future self.

Walking back on the country road... noticing the trees and flowers... breathing in the fresh air. Bring your awareness back to the room, sitting in the chair, feeling your body supported by the chair. Slowly open your eyes, stretching and yawning. Wiggling your fingers and toes... Let's take a cleansing breath, deep breath in through the nose and out of the mouth with a sigh."

Script: Imagery reprocessing for addressing grief

(*Note*: Prior to imagery reprocessing be sure to discuss with your client their beliefs about death and what is culturally appropriate and consistent with their beliefs including religious and/or spiritual beliefs. They may opt to first write a letter. This can be an important step in grieving and healing. What does the client need for closure? Discuss if they feel comfortable seeing the spirit of the person who has passed. Could they imagine them free of pain, and happy? What does the client believe happens after death? Do they believe in a soul? Would they like to do something symbolic or give them a gift? We do not know why... but for whatever reason, this person has moved on. That is their journey. Clients may opt to do imagery reprocessing while engaging in a calming hand pose—right hand on chest, and left hand on belly. Depending on the needs of the client—some may benefit from reassurance that seeing their loved-one as free, in no way diminishes their love or loyalty to that person. Releasing them is done with love, respect, and honor. Some may want to have a lasting connection where their love is eternal and can stay with them in their heart. Others may believe that they will meet again, at a later time. Thus, the imagery is tailored to individual needs, being culturally sensitive, and respectful.)

The following is an example script. Actual scripts should be created in collaboration with your client.

"Ok, let's get started with a signal breath. Take a deep breath in through the nose, hold it at the top... and slowly exhale through the mouth. Good. Feel yourself sitting in your chair, your feet on the floor, and back supported by the chair. Feel your whole body supported by the chair beneath you. Let's take another signal breath, inhale through the nose... hold it at the top... and release through the mouth. releasing any tension in the body, on the next exhale, relax your shoulders a little more, and your chest... and breathing... (extend as needed for comfort of the client).

Imagine visiting a place where (*name here*) (*the deceased person*) once was. You can see their spirit floating in the air. Imagine that you as your current age self can speak to them now. What do you want to say?.... Is there something else that you want to express?

(*Optional:* This person is on their own path, no longer bound to the experience of this worldly life. Maybe imagine them free, having no pain, and they are happy. Imagine their spirit lifting-up. Maybe they are smiling at you or telling you that they are okay. Imagine releasing them, their spirit floating upwards, going to whatever may come next. Imagine them releasing you too, letting you focus on you and your own life...)

Is there anything else you would like to say? Is there anything else you would like to do?

Bring your awareness back to the room, sitting in the chair, feeling your body supported by the chair. And taking a cleansing breath... a deep breath in through the nose and out with a sigh."

Appendix C: Client handouts

Epstein's cognitive-experiential theory: Two systems for processing information

Have you ever wanted something with your heart but knew it wasn't a good idea with your head? Dr. Seymour Epstein (2014) explains that we have two systems: a rational system and an emotional system. Both systems are important for healthy daily functioning.

Cognitive (rational) system	Experiential (emotional) system
Conscious/aware	Largely outside of awareness
Intentional	Automatic
Logical (reason oriented)	Emotional (sensation oriented)
Linear (cause and effect) & sequential (A + B = C)	Associations (guided by patterns, memories) (one thought associates to another)
Outcome oriented	Process oriented
Slow processing/delayed action	Fast processing/immediate action
Easily changes with new input (Disconfirming data influences a change of conclusion)	Resistant to change (even with disconfirming evidence, could still feel skeptical)
Requires justification, logic, evidence, reasoning (logic and facts make it true)	Self-evidently valid (I feel this way, so it must be true)

Where do you think trauma resides? If you said in the experiential/emotional system, you are correct! It is not something that can be healed through logic alone, but rather requires change in both the cognitive and experiential/emotional systems.

Epstein, S. (2014). Cognitive-experiential theory: An integrative theory of personality. New York: Oxford University Press.

Demonstrating two processing systems

Let's say you wanted to buy a car, and you researched that car A is the safest car on the market. But when you drove it, it felt like driving a tin-can. Meanwhile, you see car B drive by. You really love the way it looks, so you decide to drive it, even though it is rated lower on safety. When you drive it, it feels solid. Your heart wants car B, but your head says car A is safer. What do you do?

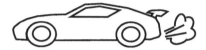

Figure C.1 Race car

Maybe you look at other factors such as price, and gas mileage. Maybe you come up with reasons to justify your decision to satisfy both your head and heart. This example demonstrates that we have two largely independent systems for how we respond to and process information. The experiential/emotional system is automatic and is typically outside our conscious awareness. It guides our everyday life from grocery shopping to conversations. Even if we think we are logical rational beings, we are highly influenced by our emotional system.

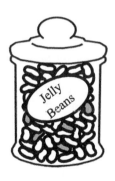

Figure C.2 Jar of jellybeans

In an experiment, students were asked to try to pick a red jellybean to win a prize. They were presented with 2 buckets of jellybeans: 10 red ones/of 100, and 1 red one/of 10. The probability of picking a red one was the same in both buckets; but, most students picked from the larger one hoping that "more" would help them win. They even picked from the larger one when there were only 9 and then 8 red ones in the larger bucket! While this behavior is illogical, it is guided by the emotional system and desire to win.

Kirkpatrick, L. A., & Epstein, S. (1992). Cognitive-experiential self-theory and subjective probability: further evidence for two conceptual systems. Journal of Personality and Social Psychology, 63(4), 534–544.

Emotion regulation skills: A quick reference guide

Emotions flow through us like water flows through a hose. They are temporary. They peak and subside. Breathe and refocus your mind, to help it pass. The following are strategies to help calm, soothe, ground yourself.

Signal breath: Take a deep breath through the nose, hold it at the top.... Then exhale through the mouth, signaling the body to relax

Cleansing breath: Take a deep breath in through the nose and exhale out with a sigh

Relaxation sandwich: Start with a signal breath and end with a cleansing breath (the sandwich can be filled with other exercises such as mindful awareness)

Grounding skills: Ground through one's senses, slow deep breathing, attention to one's feet

COPE: Cleansing breath, observation, positive self-talk, explanation

Calming hand poses: 1) Palms together, 2) hand on chest and hand on belly, 3) hand on forehead and hand on back of neck

Positive focal point: Think of something that makes you feel good—a sight, sound, song, smell, memory, prayer, saying—something to reset your mind from negative thinking or intrusive thought, something that gives you hope, and keeps you focused

Washing machine metaphor: While watching clothes in a washing machine, you stay grounded outside of the machine and observe the tumbling clothes. Similarly, stay grounded and observe having an experience like a trigger or bout of upset. Know it will end like a washing cycle. Just notice it without getting caught up in it

Katz, L. (2014). Warrior renew: Healing military sexual trauma. New York: Springer.

Coping strategies quick reference guide

When I feel anxious, tense, antsy, jittery, nervous, spacey, or unfocused I will:

1 _____
2 _____
3 _____

When I feel sad, depressed, lonely, or inadequate I will:

1 _____
2 _____
3 _____

When I feel angry, jealous, betrayed, resentful, bitter, or furious I will:

1 _____
2 _____
3 _____

When I have a nightmare or disrupted sleep, I will:

1 _____
2 _____
3 _____

When I have an intrusive thought or am reminded about my trauma I will:

1 _____
2 _____
3 _____

What is an experiential hologram?

Experiential hologram refers to a theme of experiences that re-emerge throughout a person's life. The consistent patterns repeat through time and in various contexts. Experiential holograms are formed during emotionally-charged or traumatic events. Forming these holograms may have an important adaptive function to alert people to mobilize and protect themselves in dangerous or emotionally difficult

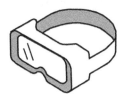

Figure C.3 irtual reality goggles

situations. They are formed from past experiences. They may feel real but it doesn't have to be that way. Just because the past was a certain way, does not mean your future has to be the same way.

Virtual reality goggles

Experiential holograms are perceptions of reality playing in the background of your mind—influencing your life. It's like wearing virtual reality goggles that filter how you anticipate, perceive, and react to life events based on your past life experiences.

Addressing the blueprints not the houses

What if you built a house from a set of blueprints and there was an issue with the house? You could try to fix the house or build a new one. But if you were using the same blueprints, then every house built from those blueprints would have a similar issue. Similarly, what if you build relationships from a relationship blueprint? Every relationship would have the same issue unless you change your relationship blueprint.

Are you responding to the present or the past?

Memories are organized or strung together through emotions. It's like plugging in a string of holiday lights. The string is the emotion, and the bulbs are all the events that are related to that same feeling. When something in the present, plugs in your string, you are likely to remember other events that are related to that feeling. For example, if you felt slighted, it may plug in a feeling of betrayal and light up memories associated with that feeling. Thus, you are not only reacting to the present but also to ALL of your past related experiences all at once.

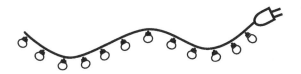

Figure C.4 A string of holiday lights

What does your future look like if you are living from the past?

If you are referencing your past when you anticipate, interpret, and respond to life circumstances, and when you make decisions, then you will be assuming things will be like your past. And if you react as if things are like your past, you will feel like it is the same. This keeps you stuck in the past. Being in the present means being open to reality as it unfolds.

"What if…" vs "What is…" thinking

We cannot *what if…* every possible scenario. If you try to anticipate danger by what if thinking you will constantly be reacting to images of fear, even when there is no actual danger. It doesn't keep you safe. It only makes you fearful. Instead, try *what is* thinking. What is happening right now? Label what is: "I am sitting right now reading. I am safe. I am breathing."

Experiential hologram discovery/mapping patterns

Think about your close relationships (romantic partners, close friends, or co-workers). What kinds of people do you attract or tend to become involved with? What disappoints you most in relationships? How do you feel when the relationship ends? The following is a writing exercise to help identify patterns adapted from *Warrior Renew* (Katz, 2014).

1 In the first column, make a list of people with whom you have had an emotionally significant or long-term relationship.
2 In the second column write a few adjectives about what qualities you liked about this person, or what attracted you to this person. *Alternate version*: Write a list of adjectives (personality qualities) that you would like in a person to date or befriend.
3 In the third column, write the things you don't like or disappointed you about these people. *Alternate version:* Write what you dislike most in people who you might date or befriend.
4 In the fourth column, write down the feelings you had at the end or shortly after your relationship ended. How did you end up feeling with this person? Even if you are still friends with the person, how did you or do you feel in these relationships? *Alternate version:* Write some of your feelings/concerns about getting into a long-term relationship or write some of your reasons why you currently are not in a relationship.

Here is an example of a completed grid:

Dylan	Independent, successful	Pre-occupied with work	Disconnected, alone
Jaden	Self-assured, was attentive to me	Bossy, self-centered	Alone, neglected
1. Relationships	*2. What attracted*	*3. What disappointed*	*4. How I felt*

Examine your list and circle words that are similar. Do you see similarities or patterns? How did you feel at the end of these relationships? Putting the information together can you summarize:

(A)   I am attracted to people who are _____.
(B)   These people turn out to be _____.
(C)   At the end of these relationships I feel _____.

Example

I am attracted to people who are: *confident, active, intelligent, and successful.*

These people turn out to be: *controlling, bossy, dishonest, and self-centered.*

At the end of these relationships, I feel: *lonely, disrespected, and invisible.*

Journal questions: Can you think of a time when you felt similar emotions to the ones you wrote in the last question (C.)? Was this feeling similar to how you felt growing up, perhaps with a parent or care-taker? Was it similar to what you observed in your parents' relationship? What do you think contributed to your feeling this way? Do you see any similarities with how you felt in adult relationships?

Interpersonal experiential hologram inventory (IEHI): A questionnaire about patterns of thoughts, feelings, and behaviors

Parenting style

Circle if any of these items describe your experiences with your parent or caregiver when you were growing up? Complete the following sentence: I **had at least one parent or primary caregiver that (was)....**

Self-focused or preoccupied	Unfair/unjust in their parenting	Was mean/ emotionally abusive
Over-involved/stifling, restrictive	Manipulated or tricked me	Valued others over me (at my expense)
Critical, judgmental	Left, or was not around, not dependable	Did not punish me when I was wrong
Did not love or care about me	Did not show me affection	Let me do whatever I wanted to
Unpredictable, inconsistent	Was difficult to please	Depended on me to take care of things
Broke promises	Was untrustworthy, lied	Created an unsafe environment
Physically hit me or sexually abused me	Disapproved of me or what I did	Did not set boundaries or restrictions

Anything else that describes your upbringing?

Private beliefs about myself

Circle the items that best describe what is characteristic of you, then pick your top 4.

I am not appreciated	I am bad/flawed	I am the only one I can depend on
I am used by others/taken advantage	I am self-doubting	I am rarely satisfied
I never feel good enough	I don't have discipline	I am unlovable
I am obligated to please others	People don't care about me	I am a failure and sabotage efforts to succeed
I am ashamed/embarrassed of myself	I am not as worthy as other people	I need to be perfect in everything I do

I am afraid to take risks	I can't trust or depend on others	I feel vulnerable in the world
I crave social attention	I am out of control	I don't need anything from anyone
I am gullible, overly trusting	I can't trust myself	I agree to things I don't want
I am forgotten/left out of social events	I am afraid of conflict	I stay in situations even when I shouldn't
I care about others more than I care about myself	I am alone in this world	I constantly worry about being safe

Anything else you privately believe about yourself?

Behaviors used to cope in the world

Circle the items that best describe what is characteristic of you, then pick your top 4.

I don't ask for help	I take responsibility for myself	I don't trust others
I do anything to please others	I fight for justice and fairness	I assume responsibility for others
I am entertaining, funny, sociable	I avoid fights/confrontation	I am skeptical of others
I like to be needed and wanted	I go out of my way to be helpful to others	I take advantage of others
I try to meet high standards	I try to "fix" others	I am pleasing and agreeable
I am trusting and loyal to others	I am seductive, sexy, and flirtatious	I break rules when I want or need to
I take charge in stressful situations	I am a perfectionist	I am ambitious and want to achieve

Anything else you do to succeed in the world? _____

Dealing with stress

What do you do when you are upset or are dealing with stress? Circle what applies to you.

| Shut down, become numb, unmotivated | Smoke, Drink alcohol, caffeine, use drugs | Relax/meditate/pray |
| Can't sit still, jittery, restless | Watch TV, play video games | Increase exercise |

Become spacey/scattered	Fight with others	Spend money, shop, gamble
Isolate, withdraw from activities	Engage in extreme sports, or take risks	Injure self (cut, burn, pierce)
Stay busy, work more, clean, organize	Seek support from others	Eat for comfort
Lose appetite, don't eat	Cut-off relationships, cancel appointments, run	Over sleep or unable to sleep

Anything else you do to deal with stress? _____

What I fear is...

Pick your top three choices and rank them from 1 to 3, where 1 is the most important to you.

Being betrayed by people I trust	Being trapped/oppressed, threatened, or Being in danger
Being criticized, rejected, judged poorly	Not being wanted
Not being loved	Being dismissed, invalidated, not believed Or taken seriously
Being unsafe/in danger	Being left/abandoned or forgotten
Being ridiculed or blamed	Something else? (Write it here)

Core violations of interpersonal experiential holograms

Below are four types of common core violations for interpersonal experiential holograms. Circle the words that best describe your life experiences and add up the number of items circled at the bottom of each column. What is most upsetting, or feels like it hits your core? Does one column stand out among the others? Endangered may include several from more than one column.

NEGLECTED	REJECTED	BETRAYED	ENDANGERED
Abandoned	Criticized	Infidelity	Unpredictable danger
Deprived	Judged	Lied to and/or manipulated	Unsafe
Emotional/physical/ or sexual neglect	Compared	Broken promises	Trapped
Ignored	Disdain/shamed	Deceived/tricked	Threatened
Dismissed	Invalidated	Unfairly blamed	Dominated
Not loved	Ostracized	Not protected	Controlled
Lack of attention Lack of self-care	Excluded/shunned	Injustice/unfairness	Emotional/ physical/ or sexual abuse
Forgotten	Put down	Taken advantage of	Gas-lighting (denial)
Overlooked	Refused	Others are disloyal	Name-calling, belittling

Write total at the bottom of each column.

Common components of interpersonal experiential holograms

Do any of these fit for you?

	Neglected	Rejected	Betrayed	Endangered
Private beliefs about myself	I'm unwanted, not important, insignificant, alone. My needs don't matter	I'm not good enough. Worries of being judged, inadequate, or failing.	I'm gullible, easily taken advantage of. People lie, are untrustworthy	I'm not safe, I'm nothing, I'm bad, out of control, others are dangerous
Compensating strategies	Be wanted: such as being helpful, funny, attentive to others, sexy, over-caring of others	Be perfect: critical of self and others, high expectations, seek perfection	Be wary: such as don't trust others. Be suspicious of others	Be safe: being submissive, or in control, avoid conflict, try to please/agree/ help others, to avoid upset
Chronic residual emotions	Depression. tired, drained, lonely	Anxiety. worried, fear of failure	Anger. resentment, paranoid	Fearful. hypervigilant, frantic, panic, overwhelmed
Motivation	To feel cared for, appreciated, attended to	To feel accepted, included, acknowledged	To feel secure, have loyalty, trust	To feel safe and secure, free from danger

Putting it together

Reflecting on the answers to previous questionnaires, what do you think best describes your life for each category?
Core violation: _____
What do you do to cope with stress? _____
Private beliefs: _____
Behaviors to cope in the world: _____
Fears: _____
What do you desire in your relationships? (e.g., loyalty or trust, to be love, appreciated, accepted, safe?) _____
Does this help clarify the components of your hologram? Do you see a theme emerging between the components? Even if one theme does not fit exactly, this might help you have an idea about what is most upsetting for you and what is important and desired.

*Core Violation (parenting style & fears):*_____
*Personal truth (beliefs about yourself):*_____
*Compensating strategy (behaviors to succeed):*_____
Avoidance strategy (when confronted with stress): _____
*Residual negative emotions:*_____
*Acquired motivation (desires):*_____

The pot on a stove

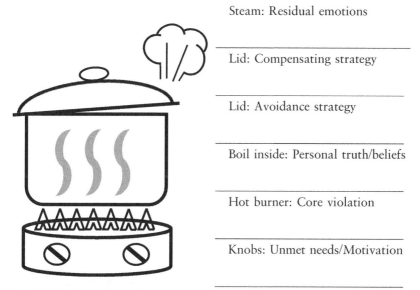

Steam: Residual emotions

_____

Lid: Compensating strategy

_____

Lid: Avoidance strategy

_____

Boil inside: Personal truth/beliefs

_____

Hot burner: Core violation

_____

Knobs: Unmet needs/Motivation

_____

Figure C.5 A pot on the stove

Metaphors for seeing context

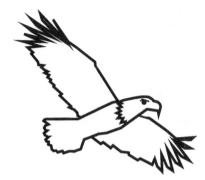

Observer vantage point

The observing eagle has a birds-eye view and can see everyone and everything involved. The eagle says, "I can see what is happening to everyone." This is the **observer vantage point**.

Figure C.6 Observing eagle

Field vantage point

The field mouse is in the field and can only see the blades of grass in front of it. The mouse says, "This is what is happening to me." This is the **field vantage point**.

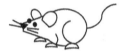

Figure C.7 Field mouse

Multiple points of view

Everyone has a point of view, agenda, and motivation.

What if you could see the same event from other people's perspective? What does each person see from their perspective?

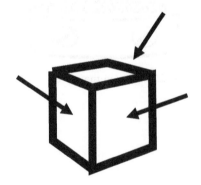

Figure C.8 Multiple view box

Age comparison (perspective of age)

Age perspective can only be seen retrospectively. When you were a younger age, you responded to life events from the field vantage point. But now that you are older, maybe you can see it a little differently? How old were you at the time of a past trauma? What do you think of someone that age now? Was there anyone else a certain age at the time that you can see differently now?

Metaphors for releasing attachment to the past

Poetic justice

When you think about the past are you disturbed because of a lack of justice, lack of closure, or feeling that the person who did something terribly wrong got away with it without consequences? This would make anyone angry! Why wouldn't it? It's unfair, immoral, likely illegal, and just very, very wrong. You have every right to be angry. However, anger takes a toll on one's mind and body, robbing a sense of joy and happiness. And that's not fair, either.

Poetic justice may be a way to disengage from the anger, hurt, and aggravation. Poetic justice is this: Somehow, somewhere, someway, people reap natural consequences of their own behavior. They will create it for themselves, eventually. You don't need to waste your precious life worrying about them, because somehow, somewhere, someway, justice will be served. *This frees you to focus on moving forward in your life.*

The blue pen

Imagine you are holding a blue pen. It is not red, or yellow... it is blue. You may be angry or hurt about it. You may have deserved a different pen. You may wake-up every morning in disbelief, resisting it, and may even throw it against the wall. Regardless of your feelings towards it, the pen is still blue. You cannot change the color of the pen, just like you cannot change the past.

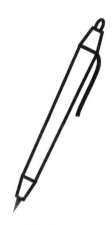

Being angry at your past for wanting it to be different is like wanting the pen to change colors. It is blue and the past is the past. Acknowledge that it was awful and should never have happened–but it did.

Figure C.9 A blue pen

Once you can take ownership of what is, it frees you from spending your energy on something that keeps you stuck in upset. It just is. This can help empower you to be present and move forward from here.

Writing letters

Writing letters is a way to gather your thoughts and express yourself to someone else or to your younger self. Think of who you would like to write the letter to. Imagine you are you, at your current age, being able to have a healing conversation. This is not used to warn or berate the person, but rather a conversation to help you get completion or peace. What do you need to say, what does the other person need to hear? What would bring you healing, or closure? Maybe sharing your new understanding or offering compassion. Two examples are:.

Letter to your younger self. In this letter, you can share what you know now as your current-age self to your younger self. Perhaps express that it wasn't the younger self's fault or shed some light about context. Maybe offer something that the younger self would appreciate. Is there anything else you would want to say? Imagine your younger self receiving your words.

Letter to your future self. Imagine meeting your future self. What would you want to say and what do you think your future self would want to tell you now?

You can write more than one letter, such as to different ages of your younger self, or to your future self, or anyone else, for the purpose of closure and healing. These are not letters to be sent in the mail to anyone. Rather they are personal for your own healing.

Figure C.10 A letter

Imagery reprocessing: Visiting your younger self

Imagery reprocessing is a technique where you, as your current-age self, imagines visiting your younger self. It is an opportunity to offer healing or compassion to your younger self.

What would you like to say? Examples are: "It's not your fault," "you are safe now," "I will always be here for you," "you are a great kid," "you matter so much."

What would you do? Examples are: take your younger self to a safe place, hold younger self in your heart, give younger self a big hug, give younger self a present, give younger self a symbol as a reminder of being ok and loved.

The imagery is intended to be gentle, and safe.

Do you know who you would like to visit? _____

Where is your younger self? _____

Do you know what you want to say or do? _____

Do not revisit a time of trauma, but rather a neutral time where you can talk to your younger self.

The process begins with relaxation, as this helps with the ability to use imagery then your therapist will guide you through a nature scene. The therapist leading the imagery will pause and check to make sure you are ready to proceed. When you are ready, imagine opening a door and seeing your younger self. This is when you will deliver your message. When you are done, you'll be guided back to the here and now.

Throughout the imagery, you remain as your current-age self and see your younger self using the observer vantage point. (You do not re-experience being your younger self.) The observer vantage point helps you see context while distancing from re-experiencing uncomfortable emotions or sensations. You will be trained on how to use the observer vantage point.

Imagery reprocessing: Surviving a near-death or dangerous event

Imagery reprocessing is a technique where you, as your current-age self, imagines visiting your younger self. In this case, your younger self who was in a near-death or dangerous situation. This could be due to a medical trauma, surviving being a victim of a crime, assault, attack, surviving a car or motorcycle accident, or natural or other disaster. At the time you were not sure you were going to make it, but now you know, you survived. Perhaps whisper in your younger self's ear— "You're going to survive this, and be alright."

What would you like to say? Examples are: "You are going to make it." "You are going to be okay." "I'm here to tell you, it's going to be alright." "Breathe. Release all the fear, you are safe now." "I'm here for you, and will take care of you."

What would you do? Examples are: Give your younger self a hug or hold your younger self's hand. Give your younger self a symbol as a reminder of being okay and safe. The imagery is intended to be gentle, and safe.

Do you know who you would like to visit? _____

Do you know what you want to say or do? _____

The process begins with relaxation, as this helps with the ability to use imagery then your therapist will guide you through a nature scene. The therapist leading the imagery will pause and check to make sure you are ready to proceed. When you are ready, imagine opening a door and seeing your younger self. This is when you will deliver your message. When you are done, you'll be guided back to the here and now.

Throughout the imagery, you remain you, as your current-age self and see your younger self using the observer vantage point. (You do not re-experience being your younger self.) The observer vantage point helps you see your younger self while distancing from re-experiencing uncomfortable emotions or sensations. You will be trained on how to use the observer vantage point.

Imagery reprocessing: Visiting someone who has died

Imagery reprocessing is a technique where you, as your current-age self, imagines visiting someone from your past, in this case, someone who has died. Maybe this person left abruptly or in a traumatic way. Maybe you witnessed the situation and could not stop or change the outcome. Complicated grief can linger for many years. It happens when there is lack of closure and feeling stuck mourning the life of someone who has passed.

Letter to someone who has died. You may opt to first write a letter as this can be an important step in grieving and healing. What do you want to say to get closure? Is there something that you want to express? Perhaps, see them in spirit form. Maybe imagine them without pain, happy, and free. What do you believe happens after death? Do you believe in a soul? There are things we do not know, but we do know, that for whatever reason, this person has moved on. That is their journey. Can you release them with love, respect, and honor?

If you can imagine speaking to them now, what would you want to say? Is there something perhaps, they may want to say to you? Remember this person is on their own path. They are no longer bound to the experiences of this worldly life. Maybe they are smiling at you or telling you they are okay. Imagine releasing them to whatever may come next. Imagine them releasing you too, to focus on your own life.

If you could visit the person who has passed,

What would you like to say? Examples: "You are safe now…and free." "Thank you." "I will always love you." "I wish you happiness on your journey." "You are a hero."
What would you like to do? Examples: Savor a moment of connection. Give them a military salute. Imagine them surrounded by angels or light.

The process begins with relaxation, as this helps with the ability to use imagery. Your therapist will guide you and check-in to make sure you are ready to proceed. When you are ready, imagine seeing the person who has deceased. This is when you will deliver your message. When you are done, you'll be guided back to the here and now. Throughout the imagery, you remain your current-age self using the observer vantage point.

Five questions to keep you in the present and out of a holographic trap!

1. What am I feeling?

_____

_____

_____

2. Have I felt this way before?

_____

_____

_____

3. Am I currently responding to a present situation or to something from the past?

_____

_____

_____

4. If I am responding to something unique to this situation, how can I best respond?

_____

_____

_____

5. If I am responding to something from the past, then how can I make it different this time?

_____

_____

_____

Post-trauma growth

Mining golden nuggets along your path

Going through trauma is horrific and nothing will diminish that. Maybe now you see a path of healing and a better future to come. From the observer vantage point, reflecting on your life and all that you have been through, could there be a golden nugget or two waiting for you?

Reflection: Consider is there something you might have gained from having lived through a traumatic experience? How might you have grown or changed in positive ways? Maybe realizing that you are stronger in ways that you might not have ever anticipated? Through grieving what you have lost, sometimes you may discover something that you have found.

Living through trauma and recovery deepens one's understanding of both pain and joy. Perhaps, the experience of healing enhances a sense of appreciation, compassion, humility, or gratitude for good things in life.

1. Can you think of something positive that you have learned as a result of going through this experience? _____

_____

_____

2. How could your past, perhaps inspire you to do something positive in the future?

_____

_____

_____

Bibliography

Abrams, J. J. (2009). *Star Trek*. Paramount Pictures.

Aghajani, S., Khoshsorour, S., & Taghizadeh Hir, S. (2021). The effectiveness of holographic reprocessing therapy on cognitive flexibility and posttraumatic growth in women with breast cancer. *Journal Arak University Medical Science*, 24(1). http://jams.arakmu.ac.ir/article-1-6471-en.html.

Ainsworth, M. D. (1969). Object relations, dependency, and attachment: A theoretical review of the infant-mother relationship. *Child Development*, 40, 969–1025. http://dx.doi.org/10.2307/1127008.

Ajzen, I. (1991). The theory of planned behavior. *Organizational Behavior and Human Decision Processes*, 50, 179–211. http://dx.doi.org/10.1016/0749–5978(91)90020-T.

Akhtar, S., Justice, L. V., Loveday, C., & Conway, M. A. (2017). Switching memory perspective. *Consciousness and Cognition*, 56, 50–57. http://dx.doi.org/10.1016/j.concog.2017.10.006.

Alexander, F., & French, T. M. (1946). *Psychoanalytic therapy*. New York: Ronald Press.

Allen, J. G., & Fonagy, P. (Eds.). (2006). *The handbook of mentalization-based treatment*. John Wiley & Sons, Inc. https://doi.org/10.1002/9780470712986.

APA (American Psychiatric Association, DSM-5 Task Force) (2013). *Diagnostic and statistical manual of mental disorders: DSM-5^{TM}* (5th ed.). American Psychiatric Publishing, Inc. https://doi.org/10.1176/appi.books.9780890425596.

Arntz, A. (2012). Imagery rescripting as a therapeutic technique: Review of clinical trials, basic studies, and research . *Journal of Experimental Psychopathology*, 3(2), 189–208.

Basharpoor, S., Narimani, M., Gamari-Givev, H., Abolgasemi, A., & Molavi, P. (2011). Effect of cognitive processing therapy and holographic reprocessing on reduction of posttraumatic cognitions in students exposed to trauma. *Iran Journal Psychiatry*, 20116(4),138–144. PMID: 22952539; PMCID: PMC3395960.

Benoit, M., Bouthillier, D., Moss, E., Rousseau, C., & Brunet, A. (2010). Emotion regulation strategies as mediators of the association between level of attachment security and PTSD symptoms following trauma in adulthood. *Anxiety, Stress, and Coping*, 23(1), 101–118. https://doi.org/10.1080/.

Bhuptani, P. H., & Messman, T. L. (2022). Self-compassion and shame among rape survivors. *Journal of Interpersonal Violence*, 37(17–18), NP16575–NP16595.

Bowlby, J. (1969). *Attachment and loss*, Vol. 1, *Attachment. attachment and loss*. New York: Basic Books.

Bowlby, J. (1973). *Attachment and loss*, Vol. 2, *Separation: anxiety and anger*. New York: Basic Books.

Braun, K., & Bock, J. (2011). The experience-dependent maturation of prefronto-limbic circuits and the origin of developmental psychopathology: implications for the pathogenesis and therapy of behavioural disorders. *Developmental Medicine and Child Neurology, 53* Suppl 4, 14–18. https://doi.org/10.1111/j.1469-8749.2011.04056.x.

Bryukhovetskiy, A. (2015). Novel theory of the human brain: information-commutation basis of architecture and principles of operation. *Journal of Neurorestoratology*, 3, 39–55. https://doi.org/10.2147/JN.S75126.

Carnelley, K., & Rowe, A. (2007). Repeated priming of attachment security influences later views of self and relationships. *Personal Relationships*, 14, 307–320. https://doi.org/10.1111/j.1475-6811.2007.00156.x.

Cattaneo, L. A., Franquillo, A. C., Grecucci, A., Beccia, L., Caretti, V., & Dadomo, H. (2021). Is low heart rate variability associated with emotional dysregulation, psychopathological dimensions, and prefrontal dysfunctions? An integrative view. *Journal of Personalized Medicine*, 11(9), 872. https://doi.org/10.3390/jpm11090872.

Dagan, O., Facompré, C. R., & Bernard, K. (2018). Adult attachment representations and depressive symptoms: A meta-analysis. *Journal of Affective Disorders*, 236, 274–290. https://doi.org/10.1016/j.jad.2018.04.091.

Daneshvar, S., Basharpoor, S. & Shafiei, M. (2022). Self-compassion and cognitive flexibility in trauma-exposed individuals with and without PTSD. *Current Psychology*, 41, 2045–2052. https://doi.org/10.1007/s12144-020-00732-1.

Declercq, F., & Willemsen, J. (2006). Distress and post-traumatic stress disorders in high-risk professionals: Adult attachment style and the dimensions of anxiety and avoidance. *Clinical Psychology & Psychotherapy*, 13, 256–263. https://doi.org/10.1002/cpp.492.

de Rios, M. D. (1997). Magical Realism: A cultural intervention for traumatized Hispanic children. *Cultural Diversity and Mental Health*, 3(3), 159–170. https://doi.org/10.1037/1099-9809.3.3.159.

Derogatis, L. R. (2000). Brief Symptom Inventory-18 (BSI-18) [Database record]. APA PsycTests. https://doi.org/10.1037/t07502-000.

DeViva, J. C. (2014). Treatment utilization among OEF/OIF veterans referred for psychotherapy for PTSD. *Psychological Services*, 11(2), 179–184. https://doi.org/10.1037/a0035077.

Dhabhar, F. S. (2014). Effects of stress on immune function: the good, the bad, and the beautiful. *Immunologic Research*, 58(2–3), 193–210. https://doi.org/10.1007/s12026-014-8517-0.

Ehlers, A., & Clark, D. M. (2000). A cognitive model of posttraumatic stress disorder. *Behaviour Research and Therapy*, 38(4), 319–345. https://doi.org/10.1016/s0005-7967(99)00123-0

Ehlers, A., Clark, D. M., Dunmore, E., Jaycox, L., Meadows, E., & Foa, E. B. (1998). Predicting response to exposure treatment in PTSD: the role of mental defeat and alienation. *Journal of Traumatic Stress*, 11(3), 457–471. https://doi.org/10.1023/A:1024448511504.

Ehlers, A., Clark, D. M., Hackmann, A., McManus, F., & Fennell, M. (2005). Cognitive therapy for post-traumatic stress disorder: development and evaluation. *Behaviour Research and Therapy*, 43(4), 413–431. https://doi.org/10.1016/j.brat.2004.03.006.

Epstein, S. (1990). Cognitive-experiential self-theory. In L. A. Pervin (Ed.), *Handbook of personality: Theory and research* (pp. 165–192). New York: The Guilford Press.

Epstein, S. (2012). Cognitive-experiential self-theory: An integrative theory of personality. In H. Tennen & J. Suls (Eds.), *Handbook of psychology*, (2nd ed.), Vol. 5. *Personality section*. Hoboken, NJ: John Wiley & Sons, Inc.

Epstein, S. (2014). *Cognitive-experiential theory: An integrative theory of personality*. New York: Oxford University Press.

Epstein, S., & Epstein, M. L. (2016). An integrative theory of psychotherapy: Research and practice. *Journal of Psychotherapy Integration*, 26(2), 116–128. https://doi.org/10.1037/int0000032.

Epstein, S., & Katz, L. (1992). Coping ability, stress, productive load, and symptoms. *Journal of Personality and Social Psychology*, 62(5), 813–825. https://doi.org/10.1037//0022-3514.62.5.813

Epstein, S., & Meier, P. (1989). Constructive thinking: a broad coping variable with specific components. *Journal of Personality and Social Psychology*, 57(2), 332–350. https://doi.org/10.1037//0022-3514.57.2.332.

Epstein, S., & Pacini, R. (2001). The influence of visualization on intuitive and analytical information processing. *Imagination, Cognition and Personality*, 20(3), 195–216. https://doi.org/10.2190/G4VG-AKQP-2Q91-JQHP.

Foa, E., Hembree, E., & Rothbaum, B. O. (2007). *Prolonged exposure therapy for PTSD: emotional processing of traumatic experiences therapist guide*. Oxford University Press.

Fonagy, P. (2002). *Affect regulation mentalization, and the development of the self*. Other Press.

Fraley, R. C., Fazzari, D. A., Bonanno, G. A. and Dekel, S. (2006). Attachment and psychological adaptation in high exposure survivors of the September 11th attack on the World Trade Center. *Personality and Social Psychology Bulletin*, 32, 538–551. https://doi.org/10.1177/0146167205282741.

Garcia, H. A., Kelley, L. P., Rentz, T. O., & Lee, S. (2011). Pretreatment predictors of dropout from cognitive behavioral therapy for PTSD in Iraq and Afghanistan war veterans. *Psychological Services*, 8(1), 1–11. https://doi.org/10.1037/a0022705.

Gendlin, E. T. (n.d.). International focusing institute. http://Focusing.org. Website pages 135–137.

Gendlin, E. T. (1996). *Focusing-oriented psychotherapy: A manual of the experiential method*. Guilford Press.

Gillath, & Karantzas (2019). Attachment security priming: a systematic review. *Current Opinion in Psychology*, 25, 86–95.

Gillath, O., Selcuk, E., & Shaver, P. (2008). Moving toward a secure attachment style: Can repeated security priming help? *Social and Personality Psychology Compass*, 2, 1651–1666. https://doi.org/10.1111/j.1751-9004.2008.00120.x.

Gray, M. J., Binion, K., Amaya, S., & Litz, B. T. (2021). Adaptive disclosure: A novel evidence-based treatment for moral injury. In J. M. Currier, K. D. Drescher, & J. Nieuwsma (Eds.), *Addressing moral injury in clinical practice*. American Psychological Association, 183–201. https://doi.org/10.1037/0000204-011.

Gray, M., J., Schorr, Y., Nash, W., Lebowitz, L., Amidon, A., Lansing, A., Maglion, M., Lang, A. J., & Litz, B. T. (2012). Adaptive disclosure: An open trial of a novel exposure-based intervention for service members with combat-related psychological stress injuries. *Behavior Therapy*, 43(2), 407–415. https://doi.org/10.1016/j.beth.2011.09.001.

Griffin, D. W. and Bartholomew, K. (1994). The metaphysics of measurement: The case of adult attachment. In: K. Bartholomew & D. Perlman (Eds.), *Attachment processes in adulthood, advances in personal relationships*. London: Jessica Kingsley Publishers, 17–52.

Hackmann, A. (2011). Imagery rescripting in posttraumatic stress disorder. *Cognitive and Behavioral Practice*, 424–432.

Harlow, H. F., & Harlow, M. (1962). Social deprivation in monkeys. *Scientific American*, 207, 136–146. https://doi.org/10.1038/scientificamerican1162-136.

Hayes, S. C., Strosahl, K. D., & Wilson, K. G. (1999). *Acceptance and commitment therapy: An experiential approach to behavior change*. Guilford Press.

Hazan, C., & Shaver, P. (1987). Romantic love conceptualized as an attachment process. *Journal of Personality and Social Psychology*, 52(3), 511–524. https://doi.org/10.1037//0022-3514.52.3.511.

Hemma, G., McNab, A., & Katz, L. (2018). Efficacy of sexual trauma treatment in a substance abuse residential program for women. *Journal of Contemporary Psychotherapy*, 48 (1), 1–8, https://doi.org/10.1007/s10879–017–9365–8.

Hoge, C. W., Grossman, S. H., Auchterlonie, J. L., Riviere, L. A., Milliken, C. S., & Wilk, J. E. (2014). PTSD treatment for soldiers after combat deployment: low utilization of mental health care and reasons for dropout. *Psychiatric Services (Washington, D.C.)*, 65(8), 997–1004. https://doi.org/10.1176/appi.ps.201300307.

Holmes, E. A., Arntz, A., & Smucker, M. R. (2007). Imagery rescripting in cognitive behaviour therapy: Images, treatment techniques and outcomes. *Journal of Behavior Therapy and Experimental Psychiatry*, 38(4), 297–305.

Hudson, N., & Fraley, R. C. (2018). Moving toward greater security: The effects of repeatedly priming attachment security and anxiety. *Journal of Research in Personality*, 74, 147–157.

Janoff-Bulman, R. (1992). *Shattered assumptions*. New York: Free Press.

Kabat-Zinn, J. (1990). *Full catastrophe living: Using the wisdom of your body and mind to face stress, pain and illness*. New York: Delacorte.

Kabat-Zinn, J., Wheeler, E., Light, T., Skillings, A., Scharf, M. J., Cropley, T. G., Hosmer, D., & Bernhard, J. D. (1998). Influence of a mindfulness meditation-based stress reduction intervention on rates of skin clearing in patients with moderate to severe psoriasis undergoing phototherapy (UVB) and photochemotherapy (PUVA). *Psychosomatic Medicine*, 60(5), 625–632. https://doi.org/10.1097/00006842-199809000-00020.

Kahneman, D., Slovic, P. and Tversky, A. (1982). *Judgment under uncertainty: Heuristics and biases*. Cambridge: Cambridge University Press.

Kanninen, K. M., Punamäki, R., & Qouta, S. R. (2003). Adult attachment and emotional responses to traumatic memories among Palestinian former political prisoners. *Traumatology*, 9, 127–154.

Katz, L. S. (2001). Holographic reprocessing: A cognitive-experiential psychotherapy. *Psychotherapy: Theory, Research, Practice, Training*, 38(2), 186–197. https://doi.org/10.1037/0033-3204.38.2.186.

Katz, L. S. (2005). *Holographic reprocessing: A cognitive-experiential psychotherapy for the treatment of trauma.* New York: Brunner-Routledge.

Katz, L. (2014). *Warrior renew: Healing military sexual trauma.* New York: Springer.

Katz, L. (2016). Efficacy of Warrior Renew group therapy for female veterans who have experienced military sexual trauma. *Psychological Services,* 13(4), 364–372.

Katz, L. (2021). A single word that can change your life: The power of embracing yes, *Psychology Today.* https://www.psychologytoday.com/us/blog/healing-sexual-trauma/202109/single-word-can-change-your-life.

Katz, L., Cojucar, G., Douglas, S., & Huffman, C. (2014a). Renew: An integrative psychotherapy program for women Veterans with sexual trauma. *Journal of Contemporary Psychotherapy,* 44(3), 163–171.

Katz, L. S., Douglas, S., Zaleski, K. L., Williams, J., Huffman, C., & Cojucar, G. (2014b). Comparing holographic reprocessing and prolonged exposure for women veterans with sexual trauma: A pilot randomized trial. *Journal of Contemporary Psychotherapy,* 44, 9–19.

Katz, L., & Epstein, S. (1991). Constructive thinking and coping with laboratory-induced stress. *Journal of Personality and Social Psychology,* 61(5), 789–800. https://doi.org/10.1037//0022-3514.61.5.789.

Katz, L., Park, S., Cojucar, G., Huffman, C, & Douglas, S. (2016). Improved attachment style for female veterans who graduated Warrior Renew sexual trauma treatment. *Violence and Victims,* 31(4), 680–691.

Katz, L. S., Snetter, M. R., Robinson, A. H., Hewitt, P., & Cojucar, G. (2008). Holographic reprocessing: Empirical evidence to reduce posttraumatic cognitions in women veterans with PTSD from sexual trauma and abuse. *Psychotherapy: Theory, Research, Practice, Training,* 45(2), 186–198. https://doi.org/10.1037/0033-3204.45.2.186.

Kearney, D. J., Malte, C. A., McManus, C., Martinez, M. E., Felleman, B., & Simpson, T. L. (2013). Loving-kindness meditation for posttraumatic stress disorder: a pilot study. *Journal of Traumatic Stress,* 26(4), 426–434. https://doi.org/10.1002/jts.21832.

Kenny, L. M., Bryant, R. A., Silove, D., Creamer, M., O'Donnell, M., & McFarlane, A. C. (2009). Distant memories: A prospective study of vantage point of trauma memories. *Psychological Science,* 20(9), 1049–1052. https://doi.org/10.1111/j.1467-9280.2009.02393.x.

Kim, H. G., Cheon, E. J., Bai, D. S., Lee, Y. H., & Koo, B. H. (2018). Stress and heart rate variability: A meta-analysis and review of the literature. *Psychiatry Investigation,* 15(3), 235–245. https://doi.org/10.30773/pi.2017.08.17.

Kirkpatrick, L. A., & Epstein, S. (1992). Cognitive-experiential self-theory and subjective probability: further evidence for two conceptual systems. *Journal of Personality and Social Psychology,* 63(4), 534–544. https://doi.org/10.1037//0022-3514.63.4.534.

Kübler-Ross, E. (1970). *On death and dying.* Collier Books/Macmillan Publishing Co.

Lashley, K. S. (1929). *Brain mechanisms and intelligence: A quantitative study of injuries to the brain.* Chicago, IL: University of Chicago Press. https://doi.org/10.1037/10017-000.

Lewis, C, Roberts, N. P., Andrew, M., Starling, E., & Bisson, J. I. (2020). Psychological therapies for post-traumatic stress disorder in adults: systematic review and meta-analysis. *European Journal of Psychotraumatology*, 10;11(1), 1729633. https://doi.org/ 0.1080/20008198.2020.1729633. PMID: 32284821; PMCID: PMC7144187.

Liem, J. H., & Boudewyn, A. C. (1999). Contextualizing the effects of childhood sexual abuse on adult self and social functioning: An attachment theory perspective. *Child Abuse and Neglect*, 23, 1141–1157.

Linehan, M. M. (1993). *Cognitive-behavioral treatment of borderline personality disorder*. Guilford Press.

Littrell, J. (1998). Is the reexperience of painful emotion therapeutic? *Clinical Psychology Review*, 18(1), 71–102. https://doi.org/10.1016/s0272-7358(97)00046–00049.

Litz, B. T., Stein, N., Delaney, E., Lebowitz, L., Nash, W. P., Silva, C., & Maguen, S. (2009). Moral injury and moral repair in war veterans: a preliminary model and intervention strategy. *Clinical Psychology Review*, 29(8), 695–706. https://doi.org/ 10.1016/j.cpr.2009.07.003.

Litz, B. T., Libowitz, M. J., & Nash, W. P. (2016). *Adaptive disclosure: A new treatment for military trauma, loss, and moral injury*. New York: The Guilford Press.

Main, M., & Solomon, J. (1986). Discovery of an insecure-disorganized/disoriented attachment pattern: Procedures, findings and implications for the classification of behavior. In T. B. Brazelton & M. Yogman (Eds.), *Affective development in infancy*. Norwood, NJ: Ablex, 95–124.

McCurry, K. L., Frueh, B. C., Chiu, P. H., King-Casas, B. (2020). Opponent effects of hyperarousal and re-experiencing on affective habituation in posttraumatic stress disorder. *Biological Psychiatry: Cognitive Neuroscience and Neuroimaging*, 5(2), 203–212.

McIsaac, H. K., & Eich, E. (2002). Vantage point in episodic memory. *Psychonomic Bulletin & Review*, 9(1), 146–150. https://doi.org/10.3758/BF03196271.

McIsaac, H. K., & Eich, E. (2004). Vantage point in traumatic memory. *Psychological Science*, 15(4), 248–253. https://doi.org/10.1111/j.0956-7976.2004.00660.x.

Mehrparvar, S., Hajloo, N., Aboolghasemi, A. (2017). The effectiveness of Holographic Reprocessing Therapy on mental adjustment to cancer in women with cancer. *Studies in Medical Sciences*, 28(5), 343–352. http://umj.umsu.ac.ir/artic le-1-3923-en.html.

Mikulincer, M., & Shaver, P. R. (2008). Adult attachment and affect regulation. In J. Cassidy & P. R. Shaver (Eds.), *Handbook of attachment: Theory, research, and clinical applications* (pp. 503–531). The Guilford Press.

Mikulincer, M., & Shaver, P. R. (2016). *Attachment in adulthood: Structure, dynamics, and change* (2nd ed.). New York: Guilford Press.

Mikulincer, M., Shaver, P. R., & Berant, E. (2013). An attachment perspective on therapeutic processes and outcomes. *Journal of Personality*, 81(6), 606–616. https://doi.org/10.1111/j.1467-6494.2012.00806.x.

Mooren, N., Krans, J., Naring, G., & van Minnen, A. (2019). Vantage perspective in analogue trauma memories: An experimental study. *Cognition and Emotion*, 33, 1261–1270.

Muller, R. T., Sicoli, L. A., & Lemieux, K. E. (2000). Relationship between attachment style and posttraumatic stress symptomatology among adults who report the experience of childhood abuse. *Journal Of Traumatic Stress*, 13(2), 321–332. https://doi.org/10.1023/A:1007752719557.

Muller, R. T., & Rosenkranz, S. E. (2009). Attachment and treatment response among adults in inpatient treatment for posttraumatic stress disorder. *Psychotherapy*, 46(1), 82–96.

Najavits, L. M. (2015). The problem of dropout from "gold standard" PTSD therapies. *F1000Prime Reports*, 7, 43. https://doi.org/10.12703/P7-43.

Narimani, M., Basharpoor, S., Gamari-Givi, H., Abolgasemi, A. (2011). Effectiveness of cognitive processing therapy and holographic reprocessing on the reduction of psychological symptoms in students exposed to trauma. *Journal of Clinical Psychology*, 3(11), 41–53.

Narimani, M., Basharpoor, S., Gamarigive, H., & Abolgasemi, A. (2013). Impact of cognitive processing and holographic reprocessing on posttraumatic symptoms improvement amongst Iranian students. *Advances in Cognitive Science*, 15(2[58]), 50–62.

Neff, C.(2015).The Jaws effect: how movie narratives are used to influence policy responses to shark bites in Western Australia. *Australian Journal of Political Science*, 50(1), 114–127.

Ong, A. D., Mroczek, D. K., & Riffin, C. (2011). The health significance of positive emotions in adulthood and later life. *Social and Personality Psychology Compass*, 5(8), 538–551. https://doi.org/10.1111/j.1751-9004.2011.00370.x.

Pacini, R., & Epstein, S. (1999). The relation of rational and experiential information processing styles to personality, basic beliefs, and the ratio-bias phenomenon. *Journal of Personality and Social Psychology*, 76(6), 972–987. https://doi.org/10.1037//0022-3514.76.6.972.

Peitsch, P. (1981). *Shuffle brain: The quest for the hologramic mind*. New York: Houghton, Mifflin, Harcourt.

Pence, P., Katz, L., Huffman, C., & Cojucar, G. (2014). Delivering Integrative Restoration-yoga Nidra meditation (iRest) to women with sexual trauma at a veteran's medical center: A pilot study. *International Journal of Yoga Therapy*, No. 24, 53–62.

Phelps, J. L., Belsky, J., & Crnic, K. (1998). Earned security, daily stress, and parenting: A comparison of five alternative models. *Development and Psychopathology*, 10(1), 21–38. https://doi.org/10.1017/S0954579498001515.

Power, N., Deschenes, S. S., Ferri, F., Schmitz, N. (2020). Job strain and the incidence of heart diseases: A prospective community study in Quebec, Canada. *Journal of Psychosomatic Research*, 139, 110268. https://doi.org/10.1016/j.jpsychores.2020.110268.

Pressman, S. D., & Cohen, S. (2005). Does positive affect influence health? *Psychological Bulletin*, 131(6), 925–971. https://doi.org/10.1037/0033-2909.131.6.925.

Pribram, K. (2007). The Holonomic brain theory. *Scholarpedia*, 2(5), 2735.

Recanatesi, S., Katkov, M., Romani, S., & Tsodyks, M. (2015). Neural network model of memory retrieval. *Journal of Frontiers in Computational Neuroscience*, https://doi.org/10.3389/fncom.2015.00149.

Resick, P. A., Monson, C. M., & Chard, K. M. (2016). *Cognitive processing therapy for PTSD: A comprehensive manual*. New York: Guilford Press.

Resick, P. A., & Schnicke, M. K. (1992). Cognitive processing therapy for sexual assault victims. *Journal of Consulting and Clinical Psychology*, 60(5), 748–756. https://doi.org/10.1037/0022-006X.60.5.748.

Resick, P. A., Wachen, J. S., Dondanville, K. A., Pruiksma, K. E., Yarvis, J. S., Peterson, A. L., Mintz, J., & the STRONG STAR Consortium (2017). Effect of group vs individual cognitive processing therapy in active-duty military seeking treatment for posttraumatic stress disorder: A randomized clinical trial. *JAMA Psychiatry,*74(1), 28–36. https://doi.org/10.1001/jamapsychiatry.2016.2729.

Ricard, M., Lutz, A., & Davidson, R. J. (2014). Mind of the meditator. *Scientific American*, 311(5), 38–45. https://doi.org/10.1038/scientificamerican1114-38.

Rivinius, K. C. (2013). Sexual trauma, attachment, and dissociation in eating disorder populations. *Loma Linda University Electronic Theses, Dissertations & Projects*, 149. https://scholarsrepository.llu.edu/etd/149.

Roisman, G. L., Padrón, E., Sroufe, L. A., & Egeland, B. (2002). Earned-secure attachment status in retrospect and prospect. *Child Development*, 73(4), 1204–1219. https://doi.org/10.1111/1467-8624.00467.

Rowland, L., & Curry, O. S. (2019). A range of kindness activities boost happiness. *The Journal of Social Psychology*, 159(3), 340–343. https://doi.org/10.1080/00224545.2018.1469461.

Salehi, M., & Beshlideh, K. (2020). The effectiveness of holographic reprocessing therapy on cognitive flexibility, affective control and social adjustment on depressive patients with attempted suicide in Ilam City. *Counseling Culture and Psychotherapy*, 11(43), 183–216. https://doi.org/10.22054/qccpc.2020.50615.2338.

Salehi, M., Beshlideh, K., & Kazemzade, K. (2020). Effectiveness of holographic reprocessing therapy on cognitive emotion regulation strategies and impulsivity of women attempted suicide in Ilam City. *Quarterly Journal of Women and Society*, 11, e17192. https://doi.org/1001.1.20088566.1399.11.43.9.7.

Salehi, M., Hamid, N., & Beshlideh, K., & Arshadi, N. (2019). Comparison of the effectiveness of holographic reprocessing and dialectical behavioral therapy on cognitive flexibility and impulsivity among depressed patients with a suicide attempt in Ilam, Iran. *Journal of Ilam University of Medical Sciences*. 27(5) 1–14. https://doi.org/doi:10.29252/sjimu.27.5.1.

Schore, J. R., & Schore, A. N. (2008). Modern attachment theory: The central role of affect regulation in development and treatment. *Clinical Social Work Journal*, 36, 9–20. https://doi.org/10.1007/s10615-007-0111-7.

Seppälä, E. M., Nitschke, J. B., Tudorascu, D. L., Hayes, A., Goldstein, M. R., Nguyen, D. T., Perlman, D., & Davidson, R. J. (2014). Breathing-based meditation decreases posttraumatic stress disorder symptoms in U.S. military veterans: a randomized controlled longitudinal study. *Journal of Traumatic Stress*, 27(4), 397–405. https://doi.org/10.1002/jts.21936.

Shapiro, F. (2001). *Eye movement desensitization and reprocessing: Basic principles, protocols, and procedures* (2nd ed.). Guilford Press.

Shear, K., Monk, T., Houck, P., Melhem, N., Frank, E., Reynolds, C., & Sillowash, R. (2007). An attachment-based model of complicated grief including the role of avoidance. *European Archives of Psychiatry Clinical Neuroscience*, 257(8), 453–461. https://doi.org/10.1007/s00406-007-0745-z. PMID: 17629727; PMCID: PMC2806638.

Soller, N., Paul, J., & Mogel, A. (2008). *Yes Man*. Warner Bros. Productions.

Song, Y., Lu, H., Hu, S., Xu, M., Li, X., & Liu, J. (2015). Regulating emotion to improve physical health through the amygdala, *Social Cognitive and Affective Neuroscience*, 10(4), 523–530. https://dx.doi.org/10.1093%2Fscan%2Fnsu083.

Spielberg, S. (1975). *Jaws*. British Board of Film Classification.

Stanton, S. C., & Campbell, L. (2014). Perceived social support moderates the link between attachment anxiety and health outcomes. *PLoS ONE, 9*.

Talbot, M. (1991). *The holographic universe*. HarperCollins.

Tedeschi, R. G., & Calhoun, L. G. (1996). The Posttraumatic Growth Inventory: measuring the positive legacy of trauma. *Journal of Traumatic Stress, 9*(3), 455–471. https://doi.org/10.1007/BF02103658.

van der Kolk, B. A. (1994). The body keeps the score: memory and the evolving psychobiology of posttraumatic stress. *Harvard Review of Psychiatry, 1*(5), 253–265. https://doi.org/10.3109/10673229409017088.

van der Kolk, B. A., Burbridge, J. A., & Suzuki, J. (1997). The psychobiology of traumatic memory. Clinical implications of neuroimaging studies. *Annals of the New York Academy of Sciences, 821*, 99–113. https://doi.org/10.1111/j.1749-6632.1997.tb48272.x.

van Minnen, A., & Hagenaars, M. (2002). Fear activation and habituation patterns as early process predictors of response to prolonged exposure treatment in PTSD. *Journal of Traumatic Stress, 15*(5), 359–367. https://doi.org/10.1023/A:1020177023209.

Wallin, D. (2007). *Attachment in psychotherapy*. New York: Guilford Press.

Weathers, F. & Litz, B. & Herman, D. & Huska, J. A. & Keane, T. (1993). *The PTSD Checklist (PCL): Reliability, validity, and diagnostic utility*. Paper Presented at the Annual Convention of the International Society for Traumatic Stress Studies.

Weathers, F. W., Litz, B. T., Keane, T. M., Palmieri, P. A., Marx, B. P., & Schnurr, P. P. (2013). *The PTSD Checklist for DSM-5* (PCL-5). Scale available from the National Center for PTSD at *www.ptsd.va.gov*.

White, M. (2007). *Maps of narrative practice*. New York: Norton.

Wisco, B. E., Marx, B. P., Sloan, D. M., Gorman, K. R., Kulish, A. L., & Pineles, S. L. (2015). Self-distancing from trauma memories reduces physiological but not subjective emotional reactivity among veterans with posttraumatic stress disorder. *Clinical Psychological Science, 3*(6), 956–963. https://doi.org/10.1177/2167702614560745.

Young, J. E. (1999). *Cognitive therapy for personality disorders: A schema-focused approach* (3rd ed.). Professional Resource Press/Professional Resource Exchange.

Young, J. E., Klosko, J. S., & Weishaar, M. E. (2003). *Schema therapy: A practitioner's guide*. New York: Guilford Press. ISBN: ISBN 9781593853723.

Zakin, G., & Solomon, Z., & Neria, Y. (2003). Hardiness, attachment style, and long term psychological distress among Israeli POWs and combat veterans. *Personality and Individual Differences, 34*. https://doi.org/10.1016/S0191-8869(02)00073-00079.

Zayfert, C., Deviva, J. C., Becker, C. B., Pike, J. L., Gillock, K. L., & Hayes, S. A. (2005). Exposure utilization and completion of cognitive behavioral therapy for PTSD in a "real world" clinical practice. *Journal of Traumatic Stress, 18*(6), 637–645. https://doi.org/10.1002/jts.20072.

Index

For Product Safety Concerns and Information please contact our EU
representative GPSR@taylorandfrancis.com Taylor & Francis Verlag GmbH,
Kaufingerstraße 24, 80331 München, Germany

Printed and bound by CPI Group (UK) Ltd, Croydon, CR0 4YY
08/06/2025
01897006-0002